# LIMPING THROUGH LIFE

# Limping
# through Life

*A Farm Boy's Polio Memoir*

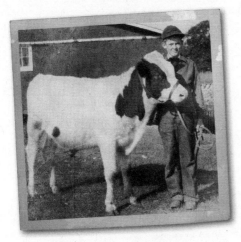

## JERRY APPS

Wisconsin Historical Society Press

Published by the Wisconsin Historical Society Press
*Publishers since 1855*

© 2013 by Jerold W. Apps

For permission to reuse material from *Limping through Life,* ISBN 978-0-87020-580-4, please access www.copyright.com or contact the Copyright Clearance Center, Inc. (CCC), 222 Rosewood Drive, Danvers, MA 01923, 978-750-8400. CCC is a not-for-profit organization that provides licenses and registration for a variety of users.

**wisconsinhistory.org**

All photos are from the author's collection unless otherwise credited.
Photographs identified with WHi or WHS are from the Society's collections; address requests to reproduce these photos to the Visual Materials Archivist at the Wisconsin Historical Society, 816 State Street, Madison, WI 53706.

Printed in Canada
Cover design by Percolator Graphic Design
Interior design and typesetting by Ryan Scheife, Mayfly Design

17  16  15  14  13      1  2  3  4  5
Library of Congress Cataloging-in-Publication Data

Apps, Jerold W., 1934-
  Limping through life : a farm boy's polio memoir / Jerry Apps.
    p. cm.
  ISBN 978-0-87020-580-4 (hardcover : alk. paper) 1. Apps, Jerold W., 1934—Health. 2. Poliomyelitis—Patients—Wisconsin—Biography. I. Title.
  RC180.2.A67 2013
  616.8350092—dc23
  [B]

                    2012032704

♾ The paper used in this publication meets the minimum requirements of the American National Standard for Information Sciences—Permanence of Paper for Printed Library Materials, ANSI Z39.48—1992.

*To Herman and Eleanor Apps, my parents, and Faith Jenks, my eighth grade teacher, who through their encouragement and caring got me through my worst days with polio.*

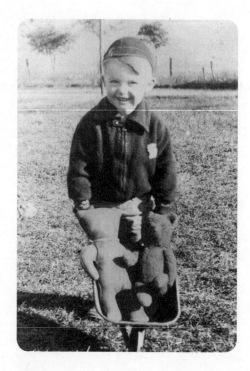

# Contents

# Preface

Polio is rarely talked about today, especially in the United States. Yet those of us who had the disease remember it all too well. In the 1940s and 1950s, before a vaccine was developed, polio dashed hopes, generated near terror in communities throughout the country, caused untold anguish for victims and their families, and dramatically changed the lives of those who contracted it.

The years just after World War II, roughly 1946 to 1955, were the peak years for polio outbreaks in this country. Wisconsin had one of its worst epidemics in 1955, when the state reported 921 cases and 134 deaths due to polio by August. The worst year for polio in the United States was 1952, when 60,000 cases were reported nationwide.[1]

Also known as poliomyelitis or infantile paralysis, polio is an infectious viral disease that most commonly attacks children, more boys than girls. Before the cause and spread of the disease were understood, many people incorrectly thought it was spread by sneezing and coughing, like many influenza viruses. Researchers ultimately

---

1. Amanda Boeker and Valerie Brandt, "Living in Fear: Northeast Wisconsin's Polio Epidemics," *Voyageur*, Winter/Spring 2007, 10.

determined that polio is caused by a virus that enters the body through the mouth and moves into the intestinal tract. The main breeding ground for the virus is the small intestine. The disease spreads from person to person by unwashed hands after using the bathroom or through contaminated food and water.

Testing began on Jonas Salk's polio vaccine in 1952. But the vaccine would not be widely available until 1955, and even after that time people lived in fear of contracting the disease. Not knowing how the disease was transmitted resulted in a near panic in some communities. Swimming pools were closed, county fairs cancelled, family picnics postponed. People feared going anywhere there was a crowd.

Today people often ask me how I got polio. I have no idea. I was the only one at my school to come down with the disease. Neither of my brothers got it—perhaps because my folks kept them away from me almost immediately after my symptoms appeared. One boy from a nearby school district had died from polio a few months before I became ill, but I had not been in contact with him. Several other children in and around my hometown of Wild Rose had polio, but I had no contact with them either.

Little did I know at the time that I contracted polio what a profound effect it would have on me for the rest of my life, both physically and emotionally. I also had no way of knowing how it would affect my brothers and my parents. Families throughout the United States lived in fear of polio throughout the late 1940s and early 1950s, and now the disease had come to our farm. I can still remember that short winter day and the chilly night when I first showed symptoms. My life would never be the same.

# 1  First Symptoms

It came in the night, unannounced and unexpected. Just as the first November snowfall can transform the landscape in only an hour or two, the events of that evening in January 1947 would change my life profoundly.

I was twelve years old and the only student in eighth grade at the Chain O' Lake School, a mile south of our Waushara County farm. My twin brothers, Donald and Darrel, were nine years old and in fourth grade at the same school. The three of us walked home that afternoon with Marvin Miller, whose farm was just south of ours, and Lyle York, who lived three-quarters of a mile beyond our place.

Snow blanketed the countryside, three feet or deeper everywhere. The snowplows that rumbled by our farm after each storm that winter had piled the snowbanks high, and walking along the snow-packed, narrow country road was like walking in a tunnel without a top. We pulled our sleds behind us. After several days of below-zero weather, the temperature had climbed into the twenties that day, and it had been a good day for sledding on the long hill west of our schoolyard, on Lizzie Hatliff's land, during recess and our noon break. There had been

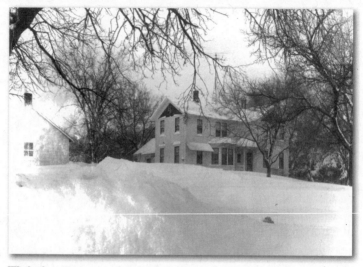

Wicked snowstorms often buried our farm, making travel impossible and chores a challenge.

lots of laughter, many spills, and several races—the kids with Flexible Flyer sleds usually won. My cheap hardware store sled served me well, but it lost most races.

At home we changed our clothes and began doing our afternoon chores. Being the oldest, I did barn chores with Pa: throwing down hay from the haymow, tossing corn silage from the silo, feeding the cows, and carrying in straw from the straw stack for bedding the animals. My brothers fed the chickens, gathered eggs, and hauled in wood for our two always-hungry woodstoves, one in the kitchen and one in the dining room. More chores waited for after supper.

We sat at our regular places around the kitchen table, Ma on one end, closest to the wood-burning cookstove, Pa at the other end, and me across from my two brothers. Just as the cows in our barn always stood in the same stall, our positions at the table never changed. The kerosene lamp had a prominent place in the middle of the big wooden table covered with a red-checked oilcloth. Its soft yellow light cast long shadows on the plain white walls of our farm kitchen. Electricity would not come to our farm until later that spring.

Our supper meal was plain but filling: fried potatoes, ham prepared in a milk-flour mixture (a smoked ham always hung on the wall of the cellar steps), steaming sauerkraut (a crock of the pungent cabbage concoction stood in the corner of the pantry), home-canned peas or corn, and applesauce or canned peaches for dessert.

Ma asked most of the questions at the supper table. "What did you do at school today? How much homework do you have? Is the teacher planning a valentine party?" She kept an eagle eye on our health, and that night she looked at me and said, "Jerold"—she always called me Jerold—"you look a little peaked," meaning I just didn't look right to her. I replied that I was a little tired from all the sledding we'd done that day, but I'd had lots of fun, and it was one of the best days I'd had that winter. She didn't say anything more.

After supper Pa and I lit our kerosene barn lanterns and headed out for the evening milking, something we did seven days a week, every week of the year. My brothers had kitchen duty, helping Ma with the dishes, making sure the wood boxes were filled, and doing other such domestic tasks. After each snowstorm we shoveled paths from the house to the barn, from the barn to the milk house, from the barn to the straw stack, from the barn to the granary, from the granary to the chicken house, from the chicken house to the house, from the house to the milk house, and from the house to the big woodpile. By the time we were finished, a maze of paths crisscrossed

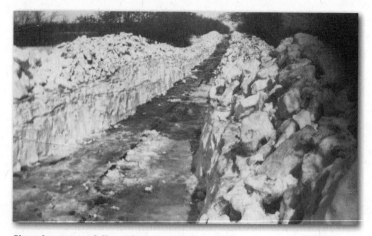

Shoveling snow followed every snowstorm. Here my dad shoveled a path so the milk truck could find its way to our farm to pick up our milk and haul it to the cheese factory.

our farmyard. I walked along the path to the barn, the lantern casting interesting shadows on the snow.

By that year we had a milking machine, a Riteway that Pa bought at the Sears store in Berlin. A temperamental Briggs and Stratton engine powered the compressor (so temperamental that sometimes it took as long to start the engine as it did to milk the cows). Pa operated the milking machine, and then he removed the machine from each cow's udders and I milked out by hand what the machine hadn't sucked out. Pa insisted on this procedure, called "stripping," because he said the last few squirts were mostly cream. The cheese factory paid for milk based on its weight and its butterfat content; the higher the butterfat level, the more money we received. At that time we milked fifteen Holsteins, and their milk's butterfat content was never as high as Pa hoped for (he wanted our milk to average around 3.5 percent butterfat). He was adamant that we gather every drop of milk the cows offered—which they seemed to do reluctantly, slapping me in the face with a wet tail or kicking at me.

With the milking finished, the oat-straw bedding rearranged under the cows one more time, and their dinner of hay pushed in front of them, we toted the ten-gallon milk cans in a wheelbarrow to the milk house a hundred or so yards from the barn, making sure to stay on the narrow, relatively snow-free path. Only then had we completed the day's work.

By eight o'clock I was back in the house and washed up from doing chores. I dug out my homework. My brothers and I did our homework in the dining room, sitting at the big table there. At the center of the table stood the kerosene-burning Aladdin lamp, which cast a much brighter and whiter light than the kerosene lamp in the kitchen. I sat with my back to the big Round Oak stove and soon was cozy warm, even a little too warm. Every half hour or so Pa stuffed another hunk of oak chunk wood, as he called the larger pieces, into the ever-hungry wood burner.

Ma noticed me nodding off, not doing much homework. "You feeling all right?" she asked.

"Just tired. Very tired," I answered.

"Why don't you go to bed? We'll find a little time tomorrow morning to finish your homework before you head off to school." Ma was a stickler about homework—and everything connected to school, including making sure we were always on time no matter what the weather or what else might be going on at home.

I lit the wick on my little kerosene bedroom lamp, the same one that my grandmother had used many years before, and made my way up the cold stairway and even colder hallway to the bedroom my brothers and I shared.

In winter Pa closed off the parlor and back room on the first floor of the house, allowing only the kitchen, the dining room, and the downstairs bedroom to receive any heat. The only upstairs bedroom that was heated, if you could call it that, was the one we boys used, situated directly over the dining room. The stovepipe from the dining room heater thrust through the bedroom floor and ended in the chimney near the bedroom's ceiling. The stovepipe provided a little heat, though not nearly enough for a big bedroom with double windows facing east. The room was as cold as I imagined an Arctic igloo to be. During much of the winter we couldn't see through the thick layer of frost covering our bedroom windows. The frost arranged itself in intricate patterns, fernlike and beautiful. To look out the window to check on the weather required first scraping off some of the frost with your fingernails, then blowing on the spot until you uncovered a peephole.

The bedroom contained a single bed, mine, and a double bed that my brothers shared. A dresser stood against one wall, and my grandmother's little rocking chair rested near where the stovepipe came through the floor. When the woodstove in the dining room burned out around midnight, a considerable chill would settle over the entire house, especially our bedroom. For sleeping we wore our long underwear, and on the coldest nights we also wore woolen socks. Ma piled each bed with homemade quilts—the result of neighborhood quilting bees—so high that once you were in bed you could barely move under the weight.

I put the kerosene lamp on the dresser, took off my thick flannel shirt and bib overalls (I wore two pair in winter), and crawled into bed. I was dead tired, about as tired as I remember ever being. I woke up several times during the night; I was too warm, and I felt the beginnings of a sore throat. Another cold coming on, I imagined. In those days I would have a cold once or twice every winter; I didn't enjoy the sore throat and runny nose, but beyond slowing me down a little, I never let a cold keep me from doing what Pa wanted me to do in the way of chores and what I enjoyed doing when the chores were done. Somehow, though, this didn't seem like a cold. My nose wasn't running. But oh, did my throat hurt, and my head was splitting when I came downstairs the following morning clutching my clothes in my arms. I usually dressed by the dining room stove, which Pa lit before he left for the barn.

My mother was working at the kitchen stove, preparing breakfast.

"How do you feel?" she asked.

"Terrible," I croaked. My throat was so sore I could hardly talk.

"Sounds like you've gotten a cold," Ma said. "You'd better stay in the house. I'll go out to the barn and tell your Pa you can't help with chores."

"Another thing," I said in almost a whisper. "My right leg hurts like the dickens."

"Probably too much sledding at school yesterday," Ma said as she pulled on her coat.

## 2    Bad News

Not only did I not do chores that morning, I did not go
to school. It would be the first day of school I had missed
since the start of the year in September. At the end of the
school year all eighth graders in Waushara County would
take a battery of tests to determine if they could graduate eighth grade and attend high school. I was already
worried about those tests—and missing school surely
wouldn't help.

Ma kept a close eye on me that day, holding the back
of her hand against my forehead every so often and staring down my throat. She poured warm water in a glass,
dumped in some salt, and told me to gargle. My throat
hurt so much I could hardly gargle, and the salt water
seemed to make things worse. My head pounded so I
could barely hold it up. Pain gripped my right knee. As
the day wore on, the pain grew worse. Ma gave me a
couple aspirins, but they didn't seem to help. She fixed
a place for me to rest on the dining room couch, which
stood against the wall closest to the kitchen and not far
from the wood-burning stove. She told me to keep covered up and brought me water every hour or so.

Pain wasn't entirely new to me. Farm kids get themselves into all sorts of situations where they get bumped and bruised. A horse steps on your foot when you're trying to harness it, or it pushes you against its stall just because you happen to be there. Your 4-H calf decides it doesn't want to learn how to lead and bounds off, dragging you along behind, desperately holding on to the rope. You run onto a bumble bee nest while you're making hay, and three or four angry bees drill into your hide. But this was a pain like I had never known before. I felt like crying, but I knew that wouldn't help—and besides, a twelve-year-old boy wasn't supposed to cry, no matter what. Crying was for city kids and girls. At times I had to bite my lip, my leg hurt so much.

When Pa came in at lunchtime, I overheard Ma telling him that I seemed to have gotten worse. She wondered if they should take me to the doctor in Wild Rose. Pa, not much for going to doctors, said we should wait until tomorrow and see if I was better.

That night I slept fitfully on the dining room couch, which Ma had made up into a bed for me. Most of the time I lay awake, hoping I would feel better in the morning, but the next morning I still felt terrible. My head pounded and my throat burned, and the pain in my right knee was now beyond anything I had ever experienced, even worse than when a cow had once kicked me square in the leg. It was obvious I would miss another day of school.

"I think we should take Jerold to see Dr. Hadden at the hospital," Ma said. Pa didn't disagree.

With a population of fewer than six hundred, Wild Rose was lucky to have a hospital, a rarity for towns that size. Dr. Hadden, a Chicago native, had vacationed in the Wild Rose area, liked the community, and started a practice and built a hospital there in 1941. (Wild Rose still has the only hospital in Waushara County.)

Ma bundled me up and, with Pa, helped me into our 1936 Plymouth, the car we'd had all through the war. My knee hurt even more when I walked. Our farm was four and a half miles west of Wild Rose, an easy drive, especially after we turned off our country road onto County Highway A, which had a hard surface and was regularly plowed free of snow.

I had never been inside the Wild Rose hospital before but had ridden past it many times. It stood on a knoll on the north side of town, not far from the cheese factory and across Highway 22 from the grist mill where we took our corn and oats to be ground into cow feed. Pa helped me into the hospital, and I slumped into a chair. Ma sat with me while he told the receptionist that he'd like Dr. Hadden to have a look at me. The hospital was a busy place, with smells unlike anything I'd encountered before—nothing like the familiar aromas of the cheese factory and grist mill, or our own barn, chicken house, and woodshed.

Soon Dr. Hadden appeared, a middle-aged, mild-mannered man wearing a white coat. "What have we here?" he asked.

"It's Jerold," Ma said. She had the kind of look on her face that she got when a cow was sick or something seemed wrong with the chicken flock. "He's got a fierce headache and sore throat, and his right leg doesn't seem to work right."

As my parents stayed behind in the waiting area, Dr. Hadden helped me into a little examination room. There I sat on a cloth-covered table and tried to explain where I hurt and when I had started hurting. Dr. Hadden looked down my throat, took my temperature, and then had me roll up my pant leg so he could look at my leg. "Hmm," was all I heard him say. But the more he examined me, the more the look on his face matched the one Ma had. A worried look.

Dr. Hadden left me for a few minutes while he went to fetch Pa and Ma from the waiting room. "What's wrong with him?" Pa asked. He was never one to beat around the bush. He wanted to know the truth of something, straight out, with no fancy language.

"I don't really know," Dr. Hadden said quietly. "It could be the start of a bad cold, but with the pain in his leg, it could be more than that."

"What do you think it is?" asked Ma.

"Well, it could be rheumatic fever. Symptoms fit: fever, painful joints, sore throat. Take him home, give him lots of liquids, and come back in a couple days if he's not better." If Dr. Hadden had any thoughts about what else might be ailing me, he didn't reveal them at the time.

On the way home, we stopped at the mercantile in Wild Rose and Ma bought some canned orange juice. At home she poured me a glass. In those days we rarely ate oranges, usually only at Christmas as a special treat. The canned juice tasted awful, not at all like what I knew a fresh orange tasted like. I suspect my high fever contributed to the bad taste—nothing tasted right to me, and I had no appetite. That afternoon Ma baked homemade bread, cut me a big slice, and spread it with butter and homemade strawberry jam. I couldn't eat it. It just didn't taste right.

I slept little that night, and in the morning I felt even worse. When I crawled off the coach, I discovered I couldn't stand up and nearly fell before catching myself on a chair. Something was dreadfully wrong with me. I couldn't bend my knee. It was frozen at a forty-five-degree bend. When Ma asked me to stand up, I held on to a chair and managed to stand, but my right knee remained bent; about the best I could do with my right leg was touch the end of my toes on the floor. I was beginning to feel really scared.

"I think we should take Jerold to see Dr. Hadden again," Ma said when Pa came in from doing the morning chores. Although they were speaking calmly, I could see deep concern in their faces. By this time even my twin brothers, Donald and Darrel, seemed concerned as well. Maybe they were worried that they would have to pick up even more of my chores, or maybe they wondered if they could catch whatever I had. They didn't say. My folks helped me pull on my Mackinaw coat, and I half hopped and half leaned on Pa as he helped me into the backseat of the Plymouth once again.

At the hospital, we waited a half hour or so before Dr. Hadden was available. The three of us sat quietly, no one saying a word. Pa stared straight ahead, the most serious look on his face I ever remember seeing. Ma looked down at her hands with a sad look on her face, every so often reaching over to put a hand on my bad leg and pat it gently, telling me with her action that everything would be okay. I must have looked scared, because that's how I felt.

"How you feeling today?" Dr. Hadden asked when he saw me.

"Not so good," I said. "My leg won't work."

Pa helped me into the examination room where I once more sat on the white table. Dr. Hadden looked down my throat, peered into my ears, took my temperature, and then had me roll up my pant leg so he could

look at my leg. The more he examined me, the more concerned he looked. He didn't say anything to me, didn't
ask any more questions, nothing.

"What's wrong with him?" Pa asked. "Whatta you
think he's got?"

"I think he's got infantile paralysis—poliomyelitis,"
Dr. Hadden said quietly.

"Oh, no," Ma said as she brought her hand to her
mouth. "Oh, no," she said again. Pa didn't say anything.
He just stood there with his red-checked wool cap in his
hand and a sorrowful look on his face—the kind of look
he got when one of his best cows died.

# 3   Recuperation

My mother and father stood silently, taking in Dr. Hadden's words. My folks knew about polio, of course, but like most people at the time, they didn't know where it came from or how it moved from person to person. They were very aware, however, that just a few months earlier a neighbor boy, Griffith Davies, had died of poliomyelitis. His mother, Vera, had lived with us when she was single and teaching at the one-room school west of us. She had been like a daughter to my parents, and the loss of her only son had affected our family deeply.

I heard Ma ask Dr. Hadden what treatment he recommended. He said there was little to do except let the disease run its course. There were a few cases of polio in the Wild Rose area, he told my parents. The hospital had installed several tank respirators, or "iron lungs," for patients afflicted with the most serious form of the disease, bulbar poliomyelitis, which attacks nerves that effect breathing and swallowing.

While I waited in the examination room, Dr. Hadden took my folks into his office and closed the door. Later I learned that Dr. Hadden didn't recommend that I be admitted to the hospital. In fact, he said I was rather lucky;

rather than contracting bulbar poliomyelitis, it appeared I had the paralytic form of polio, and in only one knee. I noticed that Ma was red-eyed when she came back. My parents didn't say a word on the ride home. I wouldn't know what they had talked about until a few days later, when Ma told me that Dr. Hadden had said I would likely never walk again—that I would likely spend the rest of my life in a wheelchair.

I don't remember much about the next few days. I was told later that I was ornery (my dad's word) and not pleasant to be around. People didn't know yet how polio was transmitted, other than that it seemed to move from person to person, and my parents thought it best that my brothers not be around me much. The twins had to take up the slack as far as my chores were concerned; Donald helped more in the barn, and Darrel took on the chores that both he and Donald had been doing before I got sick.

Slowly over the next several weeks the pain in my knee subsided, and then disappeared. But the paralysis remained. Several times each day I tried to bend my knee, but nothing I tried made any difference. My knee simply would not bend. Ma made me drink several glasses of canned juice each day, which Dr. Hadden had recommended (the canned grapefruit juice was even fouler tasting than the orange juice, and it was sour besides). Slowly my headache and sore throat disappeared, and my fever went down. And the pain in my frozen right knee slowly lessened. My appetite returned a little, but I was a pitiful sight. I had lost so much weight that Pa said, when someone asked about me, "He's just skin and bones."

As I slowly recovered, I remained trapped on the couch, feeling sorry for myself and complaining about

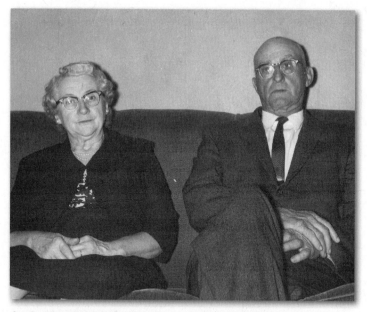

On that long drive home from the hospital, I wondered what my parents, Eleanor and Herman, were thinking about my future and about how polio would affect our family.

everything. Time passed slowly, day by day, as I listened to the ticking of the clock on the shelf just above the dining room couch.

By mid-February I began to feel much better, to the point that I was utterly bored. We had no television, of course; we didn't yet have electricity, and even if we had, TV had not yet come to our neck of the woods. Luckily, I loved to read. We had few books at home—a Bible; the Sears, Roebuck and Montgomery Ward catalogs; and some copies of *Uncle Wiggly*, a children's picture book that our mother had read to us before we started school. As I think back, both my mother and father instilled in me an appreciation for books and reading—not by encouraging me to read, but rather by not *discouraging*

me when I did. On the farm in those days, reading anything besides newspapers and the occasional magazine
was seen as a way of avoiding work. Other than the daily
newspaper and an occasional farm catalog or magazine,
neither of my parents read much. I know they never read
books. But as long as I did my chores and helped with the
work around the farm, they didn't complain when I had
my nose in a book.

The person who deserves the most credit for my
interest in reading is my first grade teacher, Theresa
Piechowski, who not only taught me how to read but
taught me the importance of reading, and the fun of it
as well. Farmers, particularly dairy farmers, were tied
to their farms, seldom traveling more than a few miles
away, as morning and evening chores beckoned seven
days a week, 365 days a year. By encouraging me to read,
Miss Piechowski opened up worlds for me. Through
books I learned about other countries and other people.
I discovered the power of a good written story. I became
acquainted with people from other places through how
they talked in dialogue. I learned about suspense and
what it takes to keep a reader reading. And perhaps most
powerfully, I could read by myself.

While I was stuck inside that winter, recuperating
from polio, my aunt Louise and aunt Arvilla brought
me books to read, wonderful books like *Bill Bolton: Flying Midshipman, Red Ryder and the Secret of Wolf Canyon,
Gene Autry and the Thief River Outlaws, Tongues of Flame,
Blondie and Dagwood's Snapshot Clue, Joyce of the Secret
Squadron: A Captain Midnight Adventure,* and *The Swiss
Family Robinson.* I read them all, book after book. In
those days, the Wild Rose Public Library was available
only to those living in the village (something about who

paid taxes to support the public library), so living in the country I did not have access to its collection. There was a small library at my school, but by the time I was an eighth grader I had read every book it held, including the very long *Uncle Tom's Cabin*. I'd read many of the library's books more than once.

Despite all the reading I was doing, I began to worry about my schooling. I had already missed several weeks of class, and the dreaded countywide eighth grade exams were looming. Ma didn't say anything, but I knew she was concerned about the county tests as well. Without telling me, she and Pa had stopped by the school to visit with the teacher, Faith Jenks, who happened to be my dad's niece. Mrs. Jenks gave them several lessons for me to work on and told them to let her know when I had finished them. She would stop by the farm to pick them up and drop off more for me to work on.

Meanwhile, Pa talked to Arnol Roberts, who ran the mercantile in Wild Rose, about my situation. Mr. Roberts gave Pa a couple of wooden orange crates. (In those days, oranges arrived in crates about three feet long and a couple feet deep, with a wooden divider in the middle.) Pa stood the crates on end about two feet apart and nailed a board across the top. I now had a desk. The dividers on each side became horizontal "shelves," providing a handy place for my schoolbooks, papers, and pencils. I thought my little desk was wonderful. Now, when I felt up to it, I could work on my lessons.

And Ma made sure that I did. No whining, no excuses: schoolwork came first. Every morning, after I dressed myself and ate breakfast, I hobbled to my makeshift desk to begin my school lessons. I walked with the aid of a kitchen chair, holding on to the back of it with both hands and pushing it forward—a clumsy, clunky way of moving, but it worked. I dragged my right leg behind me, my toes scarcely touching the floor. The chair helped me get where I was going, and then I sat on it while working at my homemade desk, which my dad had placed near a dining room window so I could look outside at the snow and cold. My folks likely couldn't afford crutches, so the old wooden, sturdy chair and I spent lots of time together.

The weeks passed, and slowly my strength returned. When I first began working on my school lessons, I couldn't work more than a half hour before I had to stop and rest. By late February I could work for as long as three hours without being overly fatigued. Mrs. Jenks started coming to the farm every day after school with new lessons for me. She would stay long enough to explain anything I didn't quite understand and answer any questions I had about the assignments.

"I'll do everything I can to help you prepare for the county exams," she said.

"I'll do the best I can," I promised. What I didn't say, but what I'm sure Mrs. Jenks already knew, was that Ma wasn't about to let me slack off, bum leg or not. Her folks pulled her out of school when she was in seventh grade to work as a maid in Wild Rose, so she never graduated from eighth grade. Pa's folks made him quit school when he was in fifth grade to work on the farm. Ma wanted her boys to have a better education than either of them had. She never said so at the time, but it was clearly something she believed in strongly. She wasn't going to let her son's gimpy leg get in the way of his education.

By early March I was able to finish all of my schoolwork in the morning. Then I could spend the afternoons reading or doing other things. Ma introduced me to

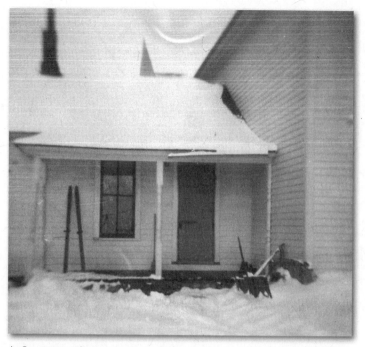

As I spent my days indoors that long winter, I spent a lot of time looking out the window.

something I'd never heard of before, spool weaving. She had Pa pound four little nails into one end of a large wooden thread spool, evenly spaced. He clipped the heads off the nails, and my little loom was ready. My aunt Edith Apps, who was a rug weaver, brought over a supply of rug-weaving warp (strong string) of various colors. I was blessed that the polio had not affected my arms or hands, so I soon caught on to the process of wrapping the heavy string around the nails, in and out, forming a long rope that slowly emerged from the hole in the bottom of the spool, like sausage oozing out of a sausage grinder. The little rope was about the width of my little finger. When I wasn't reading books, I was weaving.

Soon the rope coming out of the spool was five feet long, then ten feet long. Nobody asked me what I was going to do with my weaving. If they had, I would have answered that I didn't know. I was merely pleased to keep my fingers busy.

As I grew stronger—especially in my left leg and my arms and shoulders, strengthened from dragging my bad leg around—something else began to change. When I was hurting so bad, I didn't have time to think about much of anything other than ridding myself of the pain. As the pain began to subside, my mind focused on my studies and those county tests just a few months away. But now, with my studies on track—Mrs. Jenks said I was doing as well as any other eighth grader she had worked with and that I should be able to pass the county tests—a more terrifying thing took front and center stage in my head. I began to feel sorry for myself. I even said so to Ma once as she helped me into bed: "I'm never gonna get well."

"Not if you feel that way about it," she replied. The look on her face told me I shouldn't bring up the topic again.

As the snow began to melt in March, I could see from the dining room window above my desk that our farm fields were slowly turning from brown to green. I thought about all the things I could no longer do.

I remembered how fast I could run. I thought about the time, just last year, when we had picnicked on the Fourth of July at Silver Lake, east of Wild Rose, as we did every Independence Day. We swam in the sandy-bottomed lake and ate the big picnic lunch that Ma had prepared: potato salad, bologna sandwiches, chocolate cake, homemade dill pickles, and orange Kool-Aid.

Every year the Knights of Columbus held their July Fourth picnic at Silver Lake, with many activities going on for the kids. When the recreational director announced a footrace for ten- and eleven-year-old boys, I lined up with a dozen or so others. I remembered thinking they looked like a bunch of city kids. Not one of them wore bib overalls, which was what I wore every day of the year. A couple of the boys gave me the once over, but I didn't say anything. Wild Rose was a tourist town in those days (it still is), and I was accustomed to having city kids look at me like I was some strange kind of bird fresh off the farm (which I was).

The leader said "Go!" and I lit out as fast as I could run, like I did sometimes when I went to fetch the cows in the back pasture. I left those city boys behind and claimed the first-place prize: a can of asparagus. (Canned asparagus was special in those days.)

"Where'd you get that asparagus?" Ma asked when I returned to our picnic table under the tall pine trees.

"I won it," I said. "In a footrace."

"What footrace?"

I told her about where I'd been, and a big smile spread over her face. "You know, you were racing a bunch of Catholic boys," she told me.

"They didn't look any different than any other boys, except they dressed different," I said.

"You should probably give back the can of asparagus," Ma said. But I said no, that I'd won it fair and square. Ma tucked it away in her picnic basket, smiling from ear to ear.

These were the things I thought about as I stared out the window on those early spring days and remembered how I once could run like the wind. Now I couldn't even walk. A tremendous feeling of worthlessness began to invade my mind. It was more than feeling sorry for myself, although that was part of it. It was a feeling that took me many years to overcome. Perhaps I have yet to completely put the monster behind me.

# 4 Physical Therapy

When I realized that I would never win another footrace, that I likely would never run again, I slipped into a deep funk. Today's psychologists would probably say I was depressed, but in those days a "deep funk" described my situation well. I moped around, ate little, lost more weight, and kept at my studies only when Ma insisted—indeed, demanded—that I keep up with my schoolwork or I'd flunk eighth grade and have to take the grade over again. When I said I didn't feel like studying, she would hear none of it.

My brothers avoided me. I could understand that they might be put out. After all, they had to do my chores as well as their own. But at the same time, they were going to school every day, having fun at recess, talking with their school friends, doing all the things I wished I could do. I was not fun to be around. I had nothing to talk about, nothing to share, and I was stuck in the house, walking around with a wooden kitchen chair supporting me.

Pa didn't say much about my condition, but I knew how he felt. If I even hinted to him about feeling sorry for myself, he would have none of it. Pa was very perceptive, and I knew he was well aware that my mental state had

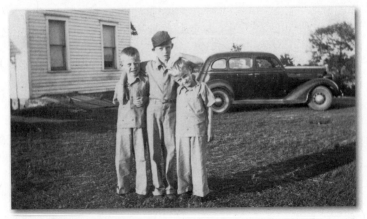

The months after I had polio were a difficult time for my brothers and me. The younger boys were doing my chores as well as theirs, and they didn't know if I would recover enough to resume working around the farm. They mostly paid no attention to me—which didn't help matters much either.

gone downhill in the last few weeks. I began comparing myself to Junior Krueger, a neighbor boy who lived a couple miles from our farm. He sat in a little wagon by County A on nice days, watching the traffic drive past, playing a guitar that had no strings. Junior Krueger couldn't walk or talk, and in my mind was about as pitiful as a person could possibly be. And he was a kid, too, fourteen years old or so. I began to imagine myself sitting in my own wagon, watching the occasional car that drove by our house or just staring off into space, worthless to myself and everyone else. When I mentioned this comparison to my parents, Pa replied, "You are not like Junior Krueger."

On a warm day in April, Pa asked if I'd like to see Stormy, my 4-H calf, a little Holstein bull that I hadn't seen since I'd gotten sick in January.

"Sure," I said. "But how am I gonna get to the barn?"

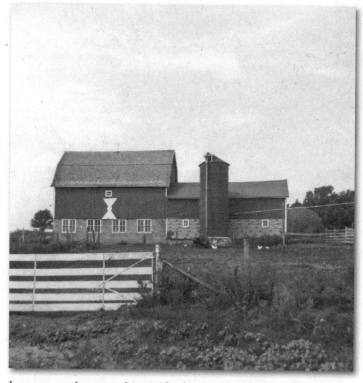

I spent many hours working in this barn on the home farm, before and after my illness.

"I'll pull you in the wagon." My brothers and I had a little red wagon that we used for everything from hauling wood from the woodpile to hauling chicken feed from the granary. Even with thoughts of Junior Krueger's wagon still stuck in my craw, if riding in the wagon was a way to get out of the house, I wouldn't protest.

Pa helped me into the wagon, once bright red but now faded and scratched from all the use and abuse it had seen. He pulled the wagon right into the barn, behind the cows. We stopped near the calf pen, where several calves rested on a bed of bright yellow straw.

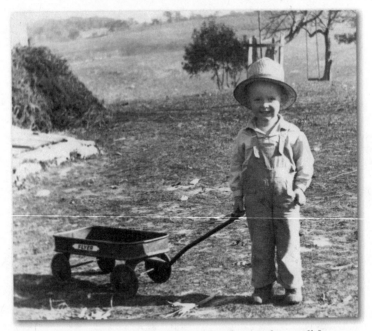

The little red wagon that had served my brothers and me well for so many years would now be my means of transport out to the barn.

"Stormy's doing well," Pa said.

I stuck my hand through the pen's wooden boards and wiggled my fingers. The calves stood up. Stormy walked over and licked my fingers. I don't know if he remembered me or not, but I was pleased that he did it.

"He's ready to be taught how to lead," Pa said. Before a calf could be entered in the county fair, it had to learn how to lead (meaning, how to be moved from place to place with a rope and halter). Calves love to run free, not to be moved around at some human's whim with a rope and halter, and teaching a calf to lead is a challenging task, even for someone with two good legs.

"How can I teach him how to lead when I can't even walk?" I said. Pa didn't say anything in reply.

I spent an hour outside in the sunshine and fresh air that day. It was the first time I had been outside since January, and it felt wonderful. My complexion was as white as the snow that had recently melted. My cheeks were sunken, and you could see my ribs sticking out if you looked close. I knew I must be the skinniest kid in the neighborhood.

The next day was again sunny and warm, as April days in Wisconsin can be. I asked Pa if he'd wheel me to my little tree nursery. In addition to my calf project, I had enrolled in the 4-H forestry project the previous year. One of the requirements was to plant one hundred seedling trees in a nursery, grow them for two or three years, and then plant them as windbreaks or in gullys and on steep hillsides that couldn't be farmed. The 4-H forestry manual explained how to make a tree nursery right down to how deep and how far apart to plant the seedling trees.

A few of the little trees had died the summer before, but most had survived. Whenever it got dry, I'd taken a five-gallon pail of water and dumped it on them. I had planted my nursery just behind the chicken house—which turned out to be a mistake. I figured it would be a handy spot, making the trees easier to take care of there. And it was. But I hadn't counted on the chickens taking a liking to my nursery and scratching out a bunch of trees. Chickens like to scratch, and I suspect they thought—if chickens think—that there might be some earthworms among my little trees. One morning I had found twenty-five little trees scratched out of the ground, their roots drying in the sun. I quickly replanted them and dumped a couple pails of water on them. I saved most of them with this quick action. Pa helped me string a length of old chicken wire around the nursery—no more chicken problem.

Now I sat in the little red wagon as Pa pulled me be-hind the chicken house to see my trees. I was concerned that the winter's snow might have done them some dam-age. But they looked just fine, a few inches taller than last summer and all bushy and green and ready to send up growth shoots for another year. I realized that my 4-H projects had come through the winter a whole lot better than I had.

By mid-April the last clumps of snow on the north side of the house melted, and spring was in the air. I spent several afternoons outside, bringing some color back to my checks and improving my appetite. But my melancholy did not go away. If anything, I felt more worthless than I had a few weeks before, when I was still cooped up in the house. My paralyzed knee had not budged, not one bit, from the day when it first froze up. Pa sometimes grabbed hold of my foot and tried to straighten out my leg, but it wouldn't straighten, and it hurt like the dickens when he did it.

Spring was a time for new growth, new ideas, new everything. And here I sat, with a bum knee and even bummer attitude. I bellyached so much about my condi-tion that the entire family was down on me. My brothers wanted nothing to do with me, and I even felt like Pa and Ma were ignoring me. And I couldn't blame them.

# 5    Tractor Challenge

Those few tastes of fresh spring air that April made me miss being outdoors all the more. Growing up on a farm, I was surrounded by nature every day, and I had already developed an abiding love of the natural world. Just a few yards from our farmhouse was a twenty-acre wood-lot stretching out to the north. There lived squirrels and rabbits, a great variety of birds, several kinds of trees, shrubs, and many species of wildflowers. Walking the mile to my country school along a seldom-traveled dusty road lined with oaks and elms provided another kind of access to nature. We were immersed in the changing of the seasons: the colors of fall, the blowing snow of winter, the muddy roads in spring, the warmth of early summer.

On Sundays my father and I, and my brothers when they were older, walked for miles exploring the woods, lakes, and fields on our farm and well beyond. In those days there were few No Trespassing signs, so we walked almost everywhere. My father had little formal educa-tion, but he knew birds and wild animals, knew their characteristics and behaviors, and could identify trees and wildflowers as well. Like a lot of farmers, he was a reasonably good predictor of weather. Pa relied on all

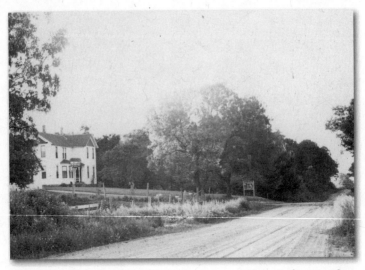

The house where I was born. A dusty country road ran in front, and nature waited just outside the back door.

of his senses when outdoors; he taught me how to listen for animal and bird calls, how to taste the difference between a blackberry and wild black raspberry, how to appreciate the smells of fallen leaves in autumn, how to see the differences between black oak, white oak, and bur oak trees. He taught me that sitting quietly in the woods on a summer afternoon when the only sound is the rustle of the breeze in the leaves and birdsong in the distance can be as pleasurable as hiking.

My dad was never much for talking, but when he said something, he meant it, and people paid attention to what he had to say. One fine, sunny day that April, he announced that it was time to work up the oat ground. The field where he planned to sow oats had been a cornfield last year; he had plowed it in the fall, so preparing it for oats was rather straightforward. This of course was not news; it clearly was time to start the spring fieldwork.

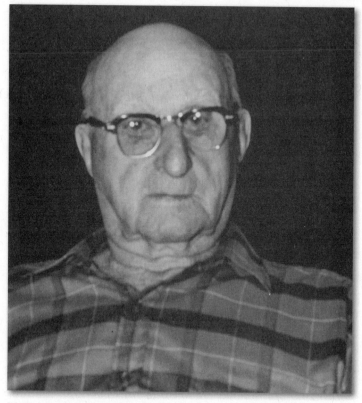

My father, Herman Apps, seen here on his ninetieth birthday. He taught me the power of remaining quiet.

But then he looked me in the eye and said, "Jerold, I want you to drive the tractor on the disc this afternoon."

I looked at him like he'd misspoken. All I could blurt out was, "What?"

"I want you to start working up the oat field out in front of the house. It's time to get the oats in the ground."

"But I can't move my knee—can't bend it at all," I said, too loudly.

"Your arms work, don't they? You can see, can't you? You can hear?"

"Yes," I muttered.

"Then you can drive the tractor on the disc. Besides, we can't have you moping around the house feeling sorry for yourself. You've been doing that since you got sick."

I didn't say anything. This was the first time I'd heard Pa say anything about my behavior. It was obvious he didn't like it, and he had plans to do something about it.

In 1946, with the war over, Pa had bought a brand new Farmall H tractor from an implement dealer in Wautoma. It was red, and it was beautiful. I had driven it several times the past year, so I knew the gear shift, how to work the clutch, how to give it more gas, and most importantly how to steer. The Farmall had two big tires in the back and two smaller ones, close together, in the front. It was a little tricky to steer, especially on soft ground. To turn, you twisted the steering wheel and at the same time applied the brake to the tractor's rear wheel on the side to which you were turning. This allowed the nonbraking wheel to power you into the turn. If you didn't do the braking, the turned front wheels merely skidded along in the direction you were headed. Pa had also bought a tandem disc, with two sections of sharp, circular blades that followed after each other, smoothing and leveling rough ground.

After we'd had our noon meal, Pa hitched the Farmall to the disc. He helped me onto the tractor seat and said he'd follow me out to the field with the team and the stone boat to pick up the stones that the disc turned up. Besides being hilly and sandy, the soil on our farm was rocky. Every spring we had to remove stones before we could plant a crop. As Pa often said, "We can depend on a crop of stones every year no matter what." He was right, as each winter's freezing and thawing brought a new bunch of stones to the surface, many fist sized, some as large as a kitchen stove.

It was a bright, cloudless day; the warm sun felt good on my back. My good left leg worked the clutch, so I had no problem putting the tractor in gear and heading off to the field, across our country road from the farmstead. My right leg, frozen at the knee, rested with my foot a few inches from the two brake pedals, one for each back wheel. The sound of the disc running along the gravel road mixed with that of the Farmall engine, which purred along without much load behind it. I hadn't driven the tractor since the previous fall, and it felt good to be doing it again. Mostly it felt good being out of the house and doing something useful for a change.

When I arrived at the field, I stopped the tractor and Pa set the disc at the angle required to work up the soil. "Take it easy when you get to the end of field," Pa said. "Ground's pretty soft, and turning may be a little tough."

I nodded, but I didn't fathom the full meaning of his words. I pushed in the clutch, put the tractor in second gear, pulled back on the gas lever, and eased out the clutch. The tractor engine groaned with the strain of the heavy machine behind it, but the big wheels turned, and we began moving across the field, the disc leveling off the furrows left from last fall's plowing. Occasionally the disc would strike a stone and make a scraping sound, but mostly all I heard was the drone of the tractor engine as we moved down the field.

I hadn't felt this good in a long time, certainly not since I'd gotten sick. The clear blue sky, the sound of the tractor and the disc, the smell of freshly worked soil, the sight of a meadowlark sitting on a fence post, and the sun on my shoulders. The field was eighty rods long, a twenty-acre field. Our farm included eighty acres on each side of the country road; the eighty acres east of the farmstead consisted of four twenty-acre fields. The field I was working was hilly, but not as hilly as some of the others in our lineup of fields.

I began to relax a little as I drove along, the disc working well, the tractor having no problems pulling it. I could see the end of the field clearly now and began planning how I would make the turn to come back for another sweep. As I neared the barbed-wire fence that marked the end of the field, I eased up on the throttle a little, listening to the engine. I had learned this from Pa: if you're pulling a heavy load, like a disc, don't slow down too much or the engine will stall. But I knew I had to slow down some because my bum knee wouldn't allow me to push on a brake pedal to properly make the turn. When I had slowed as much as I dared, I began turning the steering wheel—but nothing happened. The tractor and disc continued on toward the fence, which was only a few yards ahead of me. I tried to move my right foot onto the brake pedal, forgetting for a moment that my leg didn't work.

I turned harder on the steering wheel, but I could see the front wheels skidding in the soft dirt, coming ever closer to the wire fence. The next thing I knew, the front of the tractor hit a fence post and barbed wire flew in the air. As fast as I could react—which was not fast enough— I pushed in the clutch with my good foot, let up on the throttle, and took the tractor out of gear. Out of the corner of my eye, I could see Pa with the team at a trot coming toward me. I expected a royal chewing out. It was no fun making fence, and I'd wiped out an entire section, including breaking off a couple fence posts.

I sat on the tractor seat waiting, my head hanging down. All the good feelings I'd had just a few minutes earlier had evaporated with the sound of breaking fence posts and squeaking wire. I felt more worthless than ever.

"You hurt?" Pa called. "You hurt?"

"No, I'm not hurt," I said. "But the fence sure is."

"I see that," Pa said. He had a hint of a smile on his face. I waited for the chewing out, but none came. He helped me off the tractor, took the controls himself, and turned the machine around and pointed it in the return direction. I expected that next he would load me on the stone boat and take me home, that I'd fit into the same category as a stone that stood in the way of the spring planting.

But he didn't do that. He helped me back on the tractor, and he went back to his team. He didn't say anything—didn't say I should take it easy on the turns or watch out for wire fences. He merely went back to picking stones and left me to drive the tractor. The next turn was on firmer ground, and by slowing down to just the right speed I was able to negotiate it with minimal skidding of the front wheels. Across the field again, I faced the same predicament: soft soil, a wire fence, and a difficult turn. I noticed a spark of humor glowing somewhere deep within me. It went something like, *I've already smashed the fence, so this turn can't help but be easier.*

I slowed the tractor, began turning, and again tried to move my right foot onto the brake pedal. My knee hurt like everything when I did it, but I managed to push a little on the brake pedal. I didn't want to slam into the remnants of the broken fence. By slowing down more this time, and with just the little nudge on the brake pedal, I made the turn and was back moving in the opposite direction. After I'd turned, I noticed that Pa had been watching me the entire time. But he went back to picking stones, showing no reaction whatever.

When it was time to quit that afternoon, I drove the tractor back home. Pa helped me off the seat and into the house, where I slumped down in a chair. I was very tired, but it was a good kind of tired, the kind you feel after a solid day's work—even though it had been only an afternoon.

That evening, when the chores were done, Pa got out the Watkins horse liniment that he used for everything— horses, cows, and people. He rubbed it on my bum knee and on the muscles in my lower and upper leg. Although the liniment smelled to high heaven, it warmed up my bum knee and throttled down the pain. The warmth of the liniment felt good.

Right away the next morning, I was on the tractor again to finish working the field. With each turn, I could move my knee just a little bit more. But, oh, how it hurt. It was a different pain than I had felt before, when polio first came along. This was the hurt of sore muscles. After all, the muscles in my right leg had done little since back in January, and they were protesting fiercely.

I had the field finished by noon. Pa said I should take the afternoon off and work on my school assignments. That evening, Pa brought out the liniment again and rubbed it on my leg from my ankle to above my knee.

The next day I was on the tractor again, working in a different field. My knee bent a little more each day, until at the end of the week—although it hurt like the dickens— I could stand up with both feet on the ground. Pa kept at the liniment rubbing treatment each night, as my leg muscles continued to protest.

Now I was faced with learning how to walk again, with a right knee that was a long way from being as good as the left one. I did a slow shuffle step at first, unable to lift my right leg and dragging my foot along the ground. No longer did I need a chair to support me; I could move on my own, although it was tedious and slow. Tractor driving had been my physical therapy, providing me a very practical motivation: make my leg work, or crash into a fence.

# 6   Return to School

By the end of April I was ready to return to school, although it would be a few more weeks before I'd go back to walking the mile each way. My first week back, Pa gave me a ride each day in the Plymouth. (My mother didn't have a driver's license.) Every afternoon he stopped whatever he was doing and picked me up and drove me home. Of course, Pa also toted my brothers along on those days as well; they rather enjoyed not having to walk.

"Don't get used to this," he said. "As soon as you're walking better, you'll walk. Kids are supposed to walk to school." He knew I needed to walk to continue strengthening my bad leg.

I had missed a lot of school—two weeks in January, all of February, all of March, and two weeks in April. Going back to school felt a lot like returning after summer vacation. The other kids seemed glad to see me, and I was surely happy to see them. The school looked the same: Abraham Lincoln's and George Washington's images stared down from their locations on the front wall of the schoolroom; the big regulator clock tick-tocked just as I remembered it; model handwriting script spread out across the top of the blackboard in the front of the schoolroom, a reminder to practice our handwriting when we were finished with our other lessons.

That first morning back was chilly, so Mrs. Jenks had started a fire in the big stove that stood in back of the schoolroom. By noon she would let it go out and could even crack a couple windows to let in some fresh spring air. It was a happy day for me, the happiest I'd felt for months. I expected some of the kids would tease me about my limp and my stumbling way of walking. But no one did. Mrs. Jenks had probably laid down the law and said that nobody would tease me without risk of punishment. Or maybe no one said anything about my limp because I was in eighth grade. Country schools had a definite pecking order. Nobody messed with an eighth grader, even if he was mostly a stumblebum.

From the smallest first grader to the biggest eighth grader, everyone had duties in a country school. The schoolroom and outhouses needed daily sweeping. Someone had to carry in water from the pump house and wood from the woodshed. Waste baskets needed emptying (waste paper was saved for fire starting). Someone was in charge of keeping the woodstove going on cold days by periodically checking the stove and adding more wood. The American flag had to be put up and taken down each day. Someone had to check the mailbox to see if the mailman had left us anything (he usually didn't). First and second graders cleaned the blackboard erasers at the end of the day, the clouds of chalk dust swirling up around them. No one complained about these duties; indeed, most of the kids looked forward to doing them. Some much preferred carrying in wood to doing a page of long division problems. The problems would still have to be solved, but carrying in wood provided a nice break.

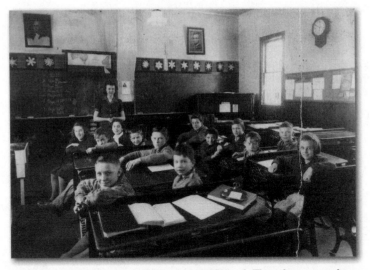

Everyone had a job to do at Chain O' Lake School. This photo was taken when I was in seventh grade and our teacher was Maxine Thompson.

The older students, from sixth through eighth, were responsible for the more important duties—at least, that's how Mrs. Jenks described them. If you did the easier tasks well—sweeping out the outhouses, cleaning the blackboard erasers—then you'd earn the right to the higher-level, more important duties. These included wood and water carrying, schoolroom sweeping, stove tending, wastebasket emptying, and the highest-level duty of all, putting up and taking down the flag.

I had a reprieve from most chores the first couple weeks I was back in school. Mrs. Jenks said I should concentrate on my studies, to continue my preparation for the eighth grade county exams. Her decision didn't sit too well with the sixth and seventh graders. Before I had gotten sick I had carried in wood, tended the stove, and put up and taken down the flag. Now, the only task I returned to was flag duty. Of course, it was mostly honorary, a task earned by doing all those other chores well over the years. A seventh grader had to give that duty back to me—not an especially happy exchange, as I recall. But flag duty required the use of only my arms, so I could still do it well, and I was proud and pleased to perform it once again as the students gathered around the flag pole every morning and afternoon.

The second week I was back in school, Pa said I should be able to walk to school, and so I did. It took me twice as long to walk that mile as it had before I got sick. So I started out well ahead of my brothers and the neighbor boys so I'd get there by the start of the school day at nine o'clock. Before I had gotten sick I could walk from home to school in about twenty minutes, depending how often I stopped to gaze at a squirrel or the neighbor's cows out on pasture or an interesting cloud formation. Now I had to leave home not long after eight to arrive at school on time.

I had always enjoyed walking to school. There was so much to see as the seasons changed and time to think about just about everything. Now I had to concentrate on walking and not tripping and falling—which I ended up doing quite often as my right foot dragged along. But even as I stumbled along our dusty country road, I enjoyed being outside again, feeling the morning sun, and smelling spring in the air. The first couple of days I was so tuckered out by the time I got to school that I couldn't do much but rest for the first hour.

My studies went well, and I quickly adjusted to the routine of the schoolroom—except for recess and noon break. While the other kids were playing anti-over; run, sheep, run; kick the can; and the other games we usually played on nice days, I could only watch. Our favorite games required running, and I could barely walk. I once again began to have those dreaded feelings of worthlessness that had overtaken me during my weeks of recovery at home.

Mrs. Jenks usually joined us outside at recess time, playing the games with us and seeming to have as much fun as the kids. "Feeling a little sorry for yourself?" she asked when she saw me watching the kids play kick the can.

I bit my lower lip, looked down at my shoes, and didn't say anything.

"I think I've got an idea for how you can participate like the rest of the kids," she said. "We're going to start softball practice next week."

I thought about what she had said for the rest of the week. What could she mean? I surely couldn't play softball; it required lots of fast running. Besides, softball was much more than merely a recess game. We played other country schools in the area, and Chain O' Lake had a reputation for having a good

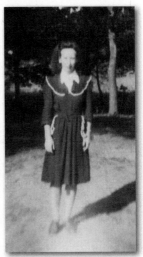

Faith Jenks, my eighth grade teacher at Chain O' Lake, helped me adjust to the school's routine after my illness.

softball team. I had been on the team since I was in the lower grades. But what could I contribute this year? Nothing. She probably had some made-up job in mind for me, like "team manager." That's what I would probably hear about the next week, when Chain O' Lake School organized its team for the spring season and began practice.

# 7   Softball

At Chain O' Lake School we played no basketball, no baseball, no football, and we had never heard of soccer. We played softball. And we played it well. We had no fancy equipment—in fact, we had no equipment at all except for a well-worn softball and a couple of wooden bats. No one used a glove, not even the catcher; no one could afford a softball glove. Besides, we farm kids, both girls and boys, had tough hands from doing chores day after day. I don't remember ever feeling a thrown or batted ball stinging my hands—it probably happened, but if you'd never used a softball glove to lessen the sting, you didn't know any better.

The softball diamond at our school was a bit unusual—I learned how unusual when we visited other schools and saw their diamonds. First of all, our diamond wasn't flat. Our schoolyard was about one acre, and when you took out the space needed for the schoolhouse, the outhouses, the pump house, and the woodshed, there wasn't a lot of real estate left for a ball diamond. It was located on a little incline just to the south of the woodshed. Big oaks grew in the outfield, several of them probably a hundred years old or more, their spreading branches providing shade for the outfielders.

When we played other schools, I also noticed that their bases usually were well-worn spots of bare ground (nobody had the fancy bases used today). At our diamond, if you made it to first you stood with your hand on a rather scraggly box elder tree rather than standing on a base. Sliding into base was a skill none of us knew, and for good reason. Who wanted to slide into a tree? To reach second base, the runner hurried uphill to touch a huge black oak tree. From second to third was downhill; third base was a white oak tree that nuzzled close to the back side of the woodshed.

Once at third base, it was downhill all the way home. Home plate wasn't a plate but merely a well-worn sandy area. You could slide into home if you wanted to, though you suffered your mother's wrath if you did—overalls got dirty enough without doing spectaculars at home plate.

The privacy fence around the boy's outhouse served as the backstop for the catcher, and a woven wire fence surrounded the schoolyard. A homerun—rather rare, because the ball had to miss the trees in the outfield— occurred when the ball dropped over the wire fence and into the dusty country road that trailed by our school.

Everyone at Chain O' Lake School was eligible to play softball, girls and boys in all grades from first to eighth. For the spring 1947 softball season, seventh graders Jim Kolka and Mildred Swendrzynski served as team captains for our practice sessions. With an elaborate system of who got first choice (hands over hands on a softball bat), Jim and Mildred selected their teams. Usually the last ones picked were the first and second graders, some kids so small they could barely shoulder a bat. During the practice sessions, the smallest players played by a different set of rules: four strikes, and halfway to first base was good enough. Older, more experienced players showed the little ones how to hold the bat, how to swing it at the ball, and how to hustle toward first base once the ball was hit, even if it rolled only a few feet toward the pitcher's mound (not really a mound but a well-worn sandy place similar to home plate).

With my bum leg, I wondered whether Jim or Mildred would select me. And I continued to wonder if Mrs. Jenks had some nonplaying softball job for me, like making sure the bats and ball were taken care of after the game. I stood watching while all the kids were selected. My brothers, Don and Darrel, in fourth grade, ended up on opposing teams—which was usually the case, as it added a little extra excitement to see them play against each other.

Finally, everyone had been selected for a team, except me. I stood there feeling awful and more than a little sorry for myself. "Jerry," Mrs. Jenks said when the kids had lined up behind their team captains and I stood there alone, "how would you like to be the pitcher for both teams? You don't have to do any running. And our school team could use a good pitcher."

I was thrilled. I would be a part of the Chain O' Lake softball team. For our interschool competitions, Mrs. Jenks would pick the best players from both practice teams, and now I thought I might have a better-than-average chance of becoming a part of the "real" team, the one that played other schools.

For a couple weeks, the practice teams played each other while I pitched. As a pitcher I wanted one of two things to happen: either striking out the batter (preferred), or making sure the batter hit the ball past me into the infield or outfield. The worst situation was a soft-hit ball that dribbled toward me, requiring that I scoop it up and throw it to first base. Several times when this happened during practice, I fell on my face trying to move quickly to grab up a ball that would have been easy for any normal pitcher to do. I felt terrible and wondered what the team would do when we played another school and I muffed what should be an easy out at first.

As for my hitting, the possibilities were clear. I either hit a homerun and hobbled my way around the bases, taking three times longer than any other player to make my way back to home plate, or I would be out at first. More times than not, I was out at first. But as the days passed, my arms and shoulders got stronger and my pitching arm a bit more accurate, and the number of homeruns I hit increased considerably. My bad leg got stronger, but it still didn't work well. I walked better, though still with a pronounced limp, but I couldn't run at all. And if I tried to move quickly in any direction, I fell down. These were not especially notable attributes for a softball player.

During those weeks I practiced pitching every night at home when my chores were done. (I was back doing most of my chores by now, and I was feeling good about being able to do them. Of course, my brothers were even happier than I was.) I marked a little square on the west end of the pump house and tried to hit inside that square with every pitch. After a week of practice, I could hit the square more than half the time—not outstanding pitching, but good enough, I hoped.

The day finally arrived for us to host another school's team at our diamond. The Willow Grove School team, accustomed to having a regular, treeless ball diamond on a flat piece of ground, was always unhappy to play at our diamond, but they came to play nevertheless.

Willow Grove was up to bat first. Our top players were ready. I was as ready as I would ever be. I took my place at the pitcher's mound, stared down at the big seventh grader, who menacingly waved his bat, and I let fly.

"Strike one!" Mrs. Jenks said. (The teachers took turns umpiring the game, standing behind the pitcher to avoid being hit by a stray pitch or foul ball.) Catcher Jim Kolka tossed the ball back to me with a big smile on his face.

I wound up and let the next one go. It was one of my slow but generally accurate pitches that arched toward home plate with little enthusiasm. The big Willow Grove seventh grader took a mighty swing at the ball, intending, I was sure, to drive it over the schoolyard fence, but he missed the ball entirely and almost fell down. Even his Willow Grove teammates chuckled at his misfortune. My Chain O' Lake teammates laughed out loud.

"Strike two!" Mrs. Jenks said. She tried to hide the grin on her face.

The Willow Creek batter, red in the face and furious at me for embarrassing him in front of his teammates, pointed the bat toward the schoolyard fence. He obviously had Babe Ruth on his mind as he stood ready for the next pitch, intent on sending the ball not just over the fence but all the way across the yard into Mac Jenks's woods.

This time I chose my fast ball, the one that Pa said was "gonna knock a hole in the pump house wall." I didn't know if he meant that as a compliment or as a warning that I shouldn't throw it so hard because I was knocking the paint off the wall. The moment the ball left my hand, I knew I'd made a mistake. The ball came in straight and true, knee high. *Crack!* I looked up to see the ball soar high overhead—not a homerun ball, but one someone in the infield would have to catch, and I wouldn't be the one to do it. Jim Kolka's brother, Dave, stood waiting in the infield for it to fall, caught it without difficulty, and the first batter was out.

The next batter, a scrawny-looking girl with pigtails, smiled at me with a silly look on her face as she stepped up to the plate. She wore a print dress, probably one her mother had made from a flour sack. But she held the bat like she knew what she was doing, and I knew I must not be put off by her silly grin.

I tossed a slow pitch that ambled its way across the plate. The scrawny girl, who looked like she didn't have enough strength to carry a pail of water, whacked the softball so hard that it fell just short of the fence. She could run like a racehorse. She reached first base and stood there touching the box elder, still grinning at me.

The next batter for Willow Grove stood at the plate. He was a little guy; I couldn't quite tell what grade he might be in. He held the bat off his shoulder and stared at me as I tried to decide what pitch to throw. The scrawny girl was still grinning when I glanced toward first base.

My pitch was a good one, right across the plate. Too good, as it turned out. The little guy's bat caught a piece of the ball, and it dribbled toward me on the ground, a few feet to my right. I went for the ball and fell down in a heap. The Willow Grove kids, not knowing about my disability, howled with laughter as the little guy easily reached first before the second baseman retrieved the ball. The smiling girl trotted up the hill to second base. I felt like I'd let my team down with my inability to run, but I did notice something: none of my Chain O' Lake teammates laughed at my misfortune.

The next batter hit another grounder, and again I fell trying to reach the ball. The Willow Grove students must have thought I was so clumsy that I kept tripping over my own feet. I'm sure it looked that way to them, as no one had told them that the Chain O' Lake pitcher couldn't run—indeed, he could hardly walk.

We lost to Willow Grove that day, 8 to 5. We had beaten them handily the previous year, and I felt awful. I told Mrs. Jenks that I had let down our team with my stumbling and falling trying to pick up ground balls.

"You'll play better," she reassured me. "You'll play better." But I wasn't sure I would ever play better. My right leg simply refused to do what I wanted it to do.

# 8    County Exams

In the midst of fretting about my athletic shortcomings, I was also worried about my academic abilities. As April came to a close, I felt the specter of the county exams hanging over my head.

Like every Wisconsin county, we had a county superintendent of schools who supervised all the one-room country schools in Waushara County. Each superintendent's office employed one or two supervising teachers, who periodically visited the schools to evaluate the teachers, check on the sanitary conditions, make sure that we all took our goiter pills (chocolaty-tasting iodine pills), and checked to see if we were following the prescribed curriculum. The supervising teachers arrived unannounced and generally unnerved the schoolteacher beyond belief. But not Mrs. Jenks. She had been teaching long enough that no county supervisor was going to make her doubt what she knew about teaching, the curriculum, keeping discipline, or anything else.

If a teacher had seventh and eighth grade students attending her school, she was especially concerned that her students passed the annual county tests. It was an obvious black mark for a teacher when students flunked these important tests.

The seventh grade tests were a breeze. You took them at your own school, and they covered only two subjects: arithmetic and reading. I had passed the seventh grade exam with no difficulty. But the eighth grade examination was considerably more challenging. It covered all academic subjects; that was challenging enough. What's more, we had to take them at the Waushara County Normal School in Wautoma, where the teachers did their training. Most Waushara County students, including me, had never seen the inside of the normal school. Of course, I had another concern: I wasn't at all sure that my home study and the work I had done since returning to school was enough to prepare me for the examination. I also had a right leg with a mind of its own. But Pa reminded me that I didn't need two good legs to take a written test.

I told Ma about my worries. "Do the best you can," she said. "That's all anyone can do." She didn't say, "I know you'll do fine." Neither did Pa. They weren't much for what educators today call "developing self-esteem." According to my folks, you got ahead if you worked hard and never quit, no matter what. If you tried your best at something and failed, that was okay. Still, I fretted and fumed and complained about having to take the exams, about how I wished my leg felt better, about how I had spoiled the softball team's chances of winning more games, and about how I generally felt awful about just about everything. Ma listened as she cooked supper on our old wood-burning cookstove, not saying anything. She'd likely gotten accustomed to my complaining and bad attitude by now.

The day of the dreaded exam arrived. I had slept little the night before, even though Ma had sent me to bed early, saying, "You've got to have your rest before you tackle the county tests." I thought, *What does she know about the county exams?* She didn't graduate from eighth grade, so she never had to take them. Pa knew nothing about the examination either. All my parents knew was that I had better pass it, or I'd be back taking eighth grade all over again. What a humiliation that would be.

It was Saturday, a beautiful, sunny day, as I remember. If I had been home, I probably would have been helping Pa prepare for corn planting. One upside to the county examination: no stones to pick on this day. It was small consolation. I'd rather be picking stones, even with my bad leg, than sitting all day taking a test.

The examination started at 8 a.m. My pa and I left home a little before seven for the twelve-mile ride to Wautoma. "Want you there in plenty of time," Pa said. My pa was never late for anything. When he told someone he'd be someplace at a given time, he was always there early. "Don't want to put anybody out by having them wait for you," he would say.

He pointed our old Plymouth down our driveway and onto the dusty country road. We drove past our herd of Holsteins out on pasture—early warm days in late April and early May had awakened the alfalfa and clover from their winter dormancy, and the pasture was a carpet of green accented by the black-and-white cows.

We drove past the cornfield, not yet planted and waiting to have its stones removed, a dirty, all-day job. On my lap I gripped my lunch bucket, in which Ma had packed two jelly sandwiches and a couple of sugar cookies. I also had three new yellow lead pencils in my hand. Pa had bought them at Stevens Drugstore in Wild Rose especially for the examination. "You gotta have a good pencil if you're gonna do well on the exam," he had said. I'd forgotten to take the pencils to school with me to sharpen them in the fancy crank pencil sharpener, so Pa had used his jackknife to put a point on the three pencils. The sharpening looked a bit rustic, but I'd tried the pencils and they worked just fine.

When we arrived at the outskirts of Wild Rose, near the Chicago and North Western Depot, we turned south on Highway 22, eight more miles to go. We were quiet as Pa sped along the highway (top speed for the Plymouth was fifty miles an hour; go faster than that and everything began shaking and shuddering). When Pa pulled into the parking area at the normal school, only a few other cars were there. I didn't have a watch, but Pa checked his prized Elgin pocket watch. "Right on time," he said. "It's a little past seven thirty."

I gathered up my lunch pail and pencils, opened the car door, and slowly limped up the sidewalk toward the school door. I glanced around to see Pa backing the Plymouth out of the parking space and heading on home. He planned to pick me up at five, when the exams were scheduled to end. I don't remember ever being more afraid, except perhaps back in January, when Dr. Hadden had said that I would likely never walk again.

I saw a sign that read County Eighth Grade Exams, with an arrow pointing toward a large room filled with tables and chairs. I walked in, carrying my lunch bucket and pencils in one hand and my cap in the other. Pa always said, "Always take off your cap when you go inside a room." I was so nervous I'd almost forgotten to do that.

A woman at the door inquired if I was there for the exams. She smiled as she spoke. I said I was and asked where I should sit. She said, "Sit anywhere you want. You're here early, so there will be a bit of a wait." I recognized a second woman holding a packet of papers as one of the supervising teachers who had visited our school from the county superintendent's office.

By five minutes to eight the room was nearly filled with eighth graders from all around Waushara County: from the Redgranite and Wautoma area, from Hancock, Coloma, and Plainfield on the west side of the county, from Poysippi, Auroraville, and Pine River to the east. From Mount Morris and Springwater and Marion townships, from Oasis, Deerfield, Richford, Dakota, and Warren townships. From Leon, Rose, Saxeville, Aurora, and Bloomfield townships. Never had I been in a room so full of scared-to-death farm kids facing a turning point in their lives.

Promptly at eight, the supervising teacher stood up to welcome us, smiled, and bid us good luck. She explained that we'd have fifty minutes for each examination, with a ten-minute break between exams and forty-five minutes to eat our lunches. "This morning you will be examined in reading, arithmetic, US history, and spelling. This afternoon we'll start with science, then geography, civics, and finally grammar."

With the help of three other women, she began passing out the examinations facedown on the table in front of us. "Do not turn over your exam until instructed to do so," the smiling woman said. Then she added, "I'm sure I don't need to remind you that you must do your own work. You may now turn over your examination papers. If you finish early, be sure to go back and check your answers and then sit quietly and wait for the next examination."

Reading was one of my favorite subjects, so I found the first exam questions fairly easy to answer. I finished a bit before most of the other students. I checked my answers once more and then sat quietly. My earlier nervousness had mostly disappeared. I remembered what Ma had said: "Do the best you can."

Arithmetic was a bit more difficult, and US history was harder still. But that was followed by spelling, which I found to be easy. When noon arrived, I quietly ate my lunch, not knowing if I could or should talk to any of the other kids. I saw a boy I recognized from our softball game against Willow Grove School. He said hi, but that's all I got out of him. He looked worried.

In the afternoon I worked my way through science (always liked the subject), geography (not difficult), civics (a bit of a challenge), and grammar (way too complicated). I turned in my last exam papers, and I was finished. It had been a long day. At quarter past five I walked out of the school, where Pa was waiting in the parking lot.

"How'd it go?" he asked as I got in the car. I must have looked beat; I was tired, and my leg ached.

"Okay, I think. They said I'll find out next week how I did."

We drove home saying little else. When we passed our cornfield, I could see the tracks left by the stone boat. I wasn't at all sorry to have missed a day of stone picking, but I wasn't looking forward to my brothers chiding me for spending a day doing sissy work. *Wait until you have to take the exams,* I thought. I was looking forward to one of Ma's big meals. She knew I must be famished after a small breakfast and only a couple of jelly sandwiches for lunch. We even had apple pie for supper, something that we seldom ate except for Sunday dinner or when relatives visited. Ma wasn't one for expressing praise in words, but she knew how to do it in other ways. Preparing my favorite meal was one of them.

# 9    Eighth Grade Graduation

As soon as I walked into the schoolroom on Monday, Mrs. Jenks asked me how the exams went. "Okay," I said. "I knew most of the answers—at least, I think I did."

"When will they let you know your grades?"

"They said they'll send them here to the school by Wednesday or Thursday."

But the letter took forever to arrive. I started checking the school mailbox on Monday, even though I knew that was too early. I checked again on Tuesday. Nothing. Again on Wednesday. Nothing.

"Do you suppose they send the grades out later for those who flunked?" I asked Mrs. Jenks when I returned from the mailbox on Wednesday.

She smiled. "I doubt that," she said. "I'm sure they send all the grade reports out at the same time. Remember," she said, "they have many tests to grade. There are lots of eighth graders this year. You told me the room at the normal school was full."

"Yes, it was," I said. "But this waiting is terrible."

"I know. But life is filled with waiting."

On Thursday when I pulled open the mailbox, I found a brown envelope from the county superintendent's office in Wautoma addressed to Mrs. Jenks, Chain O' Lake School. I hobbled into the schoolroom and up to her desk. It was recess time, and the rest of the kids were outside. She slit open the envelope and glanced at what was inside. A smile spread across her face. "You passed," she said, handing the slip of paper to me. I glanced at the grade sheet. My highest score was in science: a 99. I couldn't believe it. I did well on the spelling test, too: 96. The next best were civics, 93, and reading, 92. My worst score of all, and the grade that pulled down my average, was penmanship, a shaky 80 (75 was a passing grade). I knew I should have paid more attention to the hand-writing sample strung across the top of the blackboard at the front of the schoolroom. Although I was supposed to practice the Palmer method after I finished my other lessons, I never did. I preferred reading a book.

On the bottom of the grade sheet were the magical words: "Your diploma will be granted on Friday, June 6, at the Court House. Exercises start at 1:15 p.m. Arthur Dietz, County Superintendent." I couldn't wait for the school day to end so I could tell my mother.

My brothers didn't seem to care one way or another that I'd passed the big county test. I think mainly they were pleased that they would be attending Chain O' Lake for the next four years without having me around. Pa just smiled when I told him. Ma smiled even broader. Neither of them said congratulations or anything like that. My family was not one for passing out accolades. Doing well was expected. When you did well, it didn't require comment.

May 29, 1947, was the last day of school for the year and my last day at Chain O' Lake. As was the custom at country schools, the last day was devoted to a picnic

No. 68    Wautoma, Wis., *May 28* 194 7

*Jerold H. Apps*

*Wild Rose, Wis.*

The following are the standings earned by you at the last *8th grade* examination

Those of 65 per cent, or above are good at any examination. An average of 75 is required.

| | | |
|---|---|---|
| Reading 92 | Physiology | Manual Training |
| Penmanship 80 | Agriculture | General Science |
| Spelling 96 | Science 99 | Algebra |
| Grammar 84 | Economics | Eng. Literature |
| Arithmetic 91 | Manual | Modern History |
| Geography 89 | Library Methods | Theory and Art |
| U. S. History 90 | Domestic Science | |
| Civics 93 | American Literature | *Average 90.4* |

Your diploma will be granted on Friday, June 6, at the Court House. *Arthur Dietz*
Exercises start at 1:15 P.M.                                    County Superintendent

My grades on the county eighth grade examinations were better than I had dared to hope.

for all the schoolchildren and their parents. Everyone brought their own sandwiches and plates and silverware and a dish to pass. The school board contributed frosty metal three-gallon tubs of ice cream that rested in an insulated canvas carrying case.

There were no lessons on this last day, just a celebration—a huge picnic lunch of ham slices, potato salad, baked beans, Jell-O salads of several kinds, chocolate cake, apple pie, and much more, all laid out on the same sawhorses and wooden planks used to create the stage for our Christmas program, followed by a softball game. Several mothers brought tablecloths from home to cover the rustic planks and add a splash of color to the celebration.

Before lunch, Mrs. Jenks got everyone's attention and thanked them for coming. She said it had been a good year, and she thanked the parents for supporting her and the students during the school year. This was the eighth time I heard a teacher give this little speech, but it always made me feel good when our teacher said we had done well during the school year. Mrs. Jenks didn't mention our softball team—this had not been a winning year, mostly due to my bumbling efforts at pitcher and my propensity for falling down. Then she did say something I didn't expect. She called me over beside her and told everyone that I had handily passed my eighth grade examinations and would graduate on June 6. Everyone clapped. I'm sure I blushed, and I probably looked down at my shoes as well.

After we had eaten and everyone had sat around under the big oak trees for a half hour or so, it was time for the big softball game. This annual event was looked forward to nearly as much as the Christmas program. The fathers played against their children. We students had been playing ball since April, while our fathers hadn't played since last year's picnic. It was a sight to see.

That afternoon I pitched against a cadre of fathers who ranged from pretty good ballplayers to some who were downright awful. Even with my bum leg, I was a better player than two or three of the fathers. Those fellows swung mightily at my pitches and missed just about every time. When they did manage to hit a pitch, it flew straight up in the air and one of our infielders caught it easily. Some of the dads were very good, however, and I could do little to prevent them from hitting home runs, sometimes clear across the road and into the Jenkses' woods, where it took an outfielder ten minutes or so to find the ball.

Bob Dudley, Nita and Joyce's dad, was the fathers' team pitcher. I hate to say it, but he was a better farmer than a softball pitcher. Nearly every one of our players got hits off Bob, sometimes even home runs. I don't

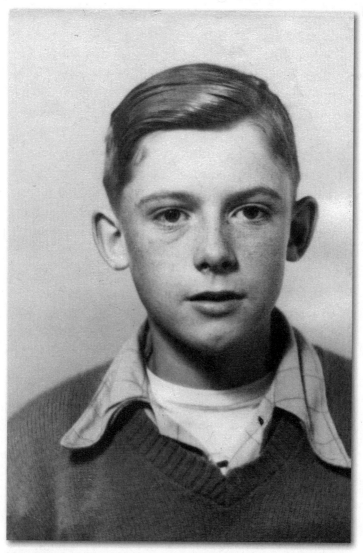

My eighth grade photo. Ready for high school?

remember the score, but our team won easily, as we had for the last several years.

But a bigger highlight than winning was getting to see our fathers play—play anything. The farmers in our school district worked all the time, and it was hard, physical work. When they weren't working, they were resting. They had neither the time nor the energy left for play—except on this last day of school each year.

My last day at Chain O' Lake was a good day. I played my favorite sport and didn't fall down once because of my bad leg. And I had managed to complete eighth grade despite having missed so many days of school during the spring term. I didn't know enough then to thank my mother for all she had done that winter to make sure I stuck to my studies. And I didn't thank Mrs. Jenks, either, for taking so much extra time to help me. I should have thanked my dad, as well, for making me get up out of my chair and begin moving. It wasn't until years later that I realized how much Ma, Pa, and Mrs. Jenks had contributed to my recovery and to helping me through eighth grade. How I wish I had known enough to thank them at the time.

On Friday, June 6, the entire family piled into our Plymouth and headed for the courthouse in Wautoma, a building that I had never been in. I wore my church pants and shirt, not my usual bib overalls that I wore every day. Pa parked the Plymouth, and we all walked into the building. The first thing I noticed when Pa pulled open the courthouse door was the smell. I'd never smelled anything like it before, not at our country school, not in any of the stores in Wild Rose, and surely not around the farm. It wasn't unpleasant, not a smell that would cause you to sneeze or your eyes to water—we had smells around the farm like that. It was simply...different. I decided to call it the courthouse smell. We spotted a sign saying Eighth Grade Graduation and pointing upstairs. Soon we were in the big courtroom, the same room where criminals were tried and sentenced. We found a seat and waited for the ceremony to begin. (Of course, we were a half hour early.) I noticed the same teachers I had seen at the examination standing at the front of the room and smiling.

I don't remember a lot about the ceremony. I limped to the front of the courtroom when my name was called, and I was handed a beautiful blue folder with my eighth grade diploma inside. When I got back to my seat, I opened the folder and read:

*Waushara County Wisconsin.*

*This is to certify that Jerold W. Apps has completed the course of study prescribed by law for the elementary schools of Wisconsin, and therefore merits this DIPLOMA which entitles the holder to admission to any high school in the state. Given at Wautoma, Wisconsin, this sixth day of June 1947.*

*Arthur Dietz, Superintendent*

When we got back home that afternoon, Pa walked into the bedroom and came back with a package that he handed to me. "This is for graduating from eighth grade," he said. I unwrapped the package, lifted the cover off a little box, and took out a beautiful pocket watch. It was a Pocket Ben, the first watch I had ever owned. Pa had already wound it and set the time. The one-dollar price tag was still on the box. Ma and Pa smiled as I admired it. Although neither of them said anything, I knew just how they felt.

# 10    Catechism

The dictionary defines *catechism* as oral instruction generally involving religious doctrine. Martin Luther said a catechism is a book of instruction in the form of questions and answers. As spring turned to the summer in 1947, I was destined to find out for myself what all these words meant.

My dad wasn't much for churchgoing, and when my brothers and I were little we were not regular churchgoers. My mother, on the other hand, had a strong church background and for a time had attended a German Lutheran parochial school near Wisconsin Rapids where only German was spoken. We did not have a German Lutheran Church in Wild Rose until 1941, so before that we occasionally attended the West Holden Lutheran Church, a Norwegian congregation, in the country near Beans Lake. Some of the Norwegians were our neighbors, and we got along well with them. But the Norwegian Lutheran Church and the German Lutheran Church were different—still are different, even after several reorganizations and consolidations.

Mother and dad liked Reverend Carl Vevle, the pastor at West Holden Lutheran Church. A few months after my twin brothers were born on January 31, 1938, Donald, the smaller of the two, became quite ill. Everyone thought he was going to die. At the time, none of us kids were baptized. On a warm July evening, Reverend Vevle drove out to our farm and baptized my twin brothers. "Might as well baptize Jerold, too," my dad had said. "As long as you're here." And so he did. I was nearly four years old at the time, and I remember the occasion well. No ceremony, no church service, just a pan of well water and the pastor. My uncle Wilbur Witt and my aunt Katherine Witt served as sponsors for all three of us. Shortly after the baptism, Donald recovered from his illness.

When St. Paul's German Lutheran Church was built in Wild Rose in 1941, we began attending there more regularly. Our pastor was Reverend Renner, a tall, thin, and very serious man. He was an old-school German Lutheran who demanded respect and mostly got it. I can't say that I ever remember him smiling. He preached a sermon in German one Sunday a month. Pa could understand only a little German, and my brothers and I knew almost no German, so the only person who would have known what was being said was our mother. Pa, never fond even of English sermons, would have nothing to do with a German one.

When I was still recuperating from polio in the summer of 1947, my mother decided I should attend catechism so I could be confirmed, something expected in all Lutheran families at the time. Instruction would be every weekday morning at St. Paul's, rain or shine, from June through August. I don't recall Ma asking me if I wanted to do it, but I'm sure she and Pa talked it over at some length. I know Pa would have preferred that I be home on the farm, but he also knew that with my bum leg I probably couldn't do a whole lot of the work that needed to be done anyway. So four other kids and I found ourselves in Reverend Renner's confirmation class that summer, meeting in the church basement every morning from nine until noon.

I had never attended Sunday school, not once, so everything about the Christian religion was new to me. (I was prone to allowing my mind to wander on Sunday mornings when we attended church, as the pastor droned on and on about something that mostly floated right over my head.) In those days nobody talked about being a Christian—what mattered was whether you were a Lutheran, Methodist, Baptist, Catholic, or Presbyterian. I didn't know about other Christian religions, let alone Unitarianism, Judaism, Buddhism, Confucianism, Taoism, Islam, or Hinduism. Even if you were a Lutheran, the differences were split rather carefully. Were you a German Lutheran, a Norwegian Lutheran, a Swedish Lutheran, a Danish Lutheran, a Wisconsin Synod Lutheran? Each proclaimed its own take on the Bible and its own sense of what was necessary to find your way out of this world to the other place—heaven, you hoped. The German Lutherans were a bit uppity about their take on Lutheranism because Martin Lutheran had been a German. (They usually failed to mention that he had been a Catholic before he decided some reforms were in order.)

Pa bought me a bicycle so I could ride the four and a half miles to town and the four and a half miles back each day and he wouldn't have to drive me there and back. It was a used bike with shiny silver front and back fenders, quite a good-looking two-wheeler. But its gear system was undependable. It's tricky riding a bike on a rutted and dusty country road. It's even trickier riding uphill on a bike whose gears slip every time you stand on the pedals to get a little more power. Generally the bike and I got along fine—except on steep hills.

The Monday morning after school got out for the summer, I was on my bike and on my way to St. Paul's German Lutheran Church in Wild Rose. It was a pleasant ride, for the most part. First I pedaled by Bill Miller's place, our neighbor to the south and about a half mile away. Then it was down Miller's hill just past their farm, braking and steering carefully to avoid a spill in the loose gravel. On the bottom of the hill, at the intersection of County Highway A and our country road, our country school stood empty and alone, awaiting the start of the fall term. County A was a blacktop road: smooth surface, easy going. I pedaled past a big white sign with black lettering, Tractors with Lugs Prohibited. In those days some of the farmers owned tractors with steel wheels, with steel spikelike affairs (lugs) on the back wheels for traction. The lugs would tear up the black top.

I turned onto County A and pedaled past Mac Jenks's farm, then past Jesse DeWitt's place. The grade was slight; I relaxed into an easy pedal. My bum leg worked reasonably well on a bike, better than I'd hoped, but I still had to rely on my left leg for most of the pedaling power. I pedaled on past Paul Krueger's place, keeping a keen eye out for farm dogs that enjoyed chasing cars and bicycles. I sailed around the corner where Otto Grabelski's driveway shot up a steep hill to the left, than a quarter mile or more farther on I pedaled past John Swendrynski's farm and made another turn for the straightaway into Wild Rose, now about two and a half miles away. I cautiously pedaled past Ernest Bryen's farm—their dog sometimes chased our car, so I expected the worst. But I saw no dog this morning. John Steinke's farm came next, on the left. No dog. Then Stanton Simon's place and Etheridge's hill ahead, the paved surface making the trip not difficult at all. I passed Dewey Etheridge's farm on the right and Otto Radloff's on the left. In a few minutes I rolled into Wild Rose, turned left onto State Highway 22, and soon arrived at the church on the right, across from the lumberyard. Not a bad ride at all—much better than I had expected, although I could feel it in my bad leg.

I parked my bike in front of the church, opened the door to the basement, and limped down the stairs. There Reverend Renner greeted me and welcomed me to the confirmation class. A couple of other kids were already there.

Stern and serious, Reverend Renner was also respectful and in his own way friendly to his students. We each soon had in our hands hardcover copies of *Luther's Small Catechism,* by Martin Luther, written in AD 1529. It was 221 pages, I discovered when I quickly checked. I immediately wondered, *If this is the "small" version of the catechism, how many pages are in the "large" version?* I thought it best not to ask—at least not this early in my formal Lutheran training.

Reverend Renner marched us through the book, introducing us to its various sections. Unfortunately, by "studying" he meant memorizing. Section one was the Ten Commandments. Luther listed each and then, so there would be no misunderstanding or an alternate take on the meaning, followed each with "What does this mean?" and the answer. I considered the sixth commandment, "Thou shall not commit adultery." I had a vague idea what *adultery* meant and at the same time somehow knew that a kid shouldn't run around asking, "By the way, what's adultery?" The "What does this mean?" answer didn't help much, either. "We should fear and love God that we may lead a chaste and decent life in word and deed, and each love and honor his spouse."

What I wanted to do with most of the "What does this mean?" answers was ask, "What in the world do these words mean?" For instance, what exactly does "leading a chaste and decent life" mean? I had never run into the word *chaste* in any of the spelling tests at my country school. So I was left wondering, and more than a little curious, why Martin Luther, Reverend Renner, and even my mother would rather dance around the meaning than spit out that adultery means that some guy ran off with another guy's wife, or some such thing. That I could understand.

When we got to the Creed, sometimes known as the Apostle's Creed, I discovered that after each statement, and the "What does this mean?" discussion, more words were added to pound each point into potentially questioning young minds. The words "This is most certainly true" discouraged kids like me from even thinking of opening our mouths to question what we were reading. "This is most certainly true" rings of finality. Case closed. End of discussion. Plant the articles of the Creed and the "What does this mean?" statements in your head and have them ready for spitting back whenever asked.

During the course of that summer, we worked our way through the Ten Commandments, the Creed, the Lord's Prayer, and what Baptism was all about; we learned about (actually, memorized) such facts as how many books are in the Bible (sixty-six) and the difference between the Old Testament (thirty-nine books) and the New Testament (twenty-seven books). We learned about the differences between historical books, poetical books, prophetical books, and epistles. It was heady stuff for a twelve-year-old, especially one who was more worried about whether he'd ever be able to walk again without a limp than about doing well in his religious studies.

Each morning that I pedaled off to catechism, my brothers were envious; once again they had to do their work and some of mine too. Had they known what I had to do in St. Paul's stuffy basement each morning, I doubt they would have said much. As far as I was concerned, they'd have to find out about catechism for themselves when they got to experience it firsthand a few years later.

By the end of summer, my fellow confirmands and I had waded through a massive amount of religious material. I did learn a couple of things as we spent those mornings meeting and memorizing: first, I learned that nobody in the class recalled anyone ever flunking the confirmation examination, which would be given on a Sunday morning in front of the entire congregation. That in itself was a comforting thought. The second thing I discovered was that one of our class members (I'll call him "Joe") had a dickens of a time memorizing. It just wasn't in Joe to come up with the statements and "What does this mean?" responses. At first I felt sorry for him and wanted to help. But then as I thought about the fact that nobody ever flunked the exam, I realized that Joe, without realizing it, was setting the bar—quite low, to be sure—for the rest of us. I knew Joe wouldn't fail—and if he could pass, and I memorized as much as he did, all would be well. Of course I didn't tell my mother about my approach to prepping for the confirmation exam.

After I'd figured out what was likely to happen at exam time, I relaxed and rather enjoyed my daily bike rides to town and away from farmwork. By late August we

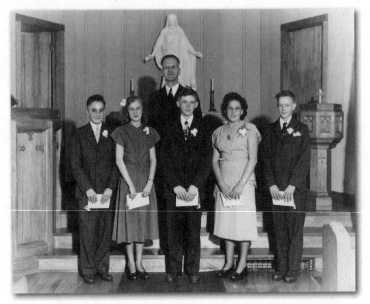

My confirmation photo from St. Paul's Lutheran Church in Wild Rose

wound up our formal instruction, and Reverend Renner planned the congregational examination for a Sunday in September.

During my last few trips to the church, I had noticed that my bike's front wheel was wobbling a little more than usual, and the back wheel was beginning to make some strange noises. When I returned from the last day of catechism, I decided to take the wheels off my bike and check what the wobbling and noise might be about. The wheel bearings fell off in my hand. The bearings in both wheels were completely worn out. I had ridden my bike into the ground that summer—it would require considerable repair before I could ride it again.

Although I was frightened out of my wits on the day of the examination, I stood up and answered my questions without difficulty, and even got the "What does this mean?" statements correct. All five of us were confirmed as new, full-fledged members of St. Paul's German Lutheran Church, eligible for communion like the adults. I had mixed feelings—I could have studied more and learned more, but on the other hand I wanted to discuss some of what I had learned, and discussion was clearly not appropriate. This was most certainly true.

Attending catechism had provided me a great benefit in addition to religious instruction: physical therapy for my leg. Riding my bike nine miles a day, up and down hills, sometimes with dogs chasing after me, sometimes with a thunderstorm threatening, strengthened my leg. I still limped, and I couldn't run, but I could walk reasonably well, and I could put in a day's work on the farm without my leg aching at day's end. My religious instruction had been extremely important, but perhaps not in the way that Ma and Reverend Renner had intended.

# 11    Stormy

When I got home from my morning catechism lessons every day that summer, I spent the afternoon working with Stormy, my little bull Holstein calf, continuing the training we had started in April. Stormy had been born on a snowy night the previous winter to one of Pa's best cows. My father sold calves of lesser quality than Stormy for veal. But every year we kept one or two good-quality bull calves and raised them to sell to other farmers for breeding purposes, providing our farm some income beyond the sale of milk from our small dairy herd.

Pa had told me the previous winter that Stormy could be my 4-H calf, and as payment for my summer work on the farm, I could keep the money earned from selling Stormy in the fall. Of course, by June much had changed for me since Pa had made me that offer. I didn't know if the deal still stood—and I didn't ask. Pa didn't bring it up as I limped my way through my barn chores and worked with Stormy each afternoon.

Stormy was a strong-willed creature with a mind of his own. Right from the beginning he had done pretty much whatever he wanted to do, and by summer he had grown into a strong, rambunctious little bull. In order

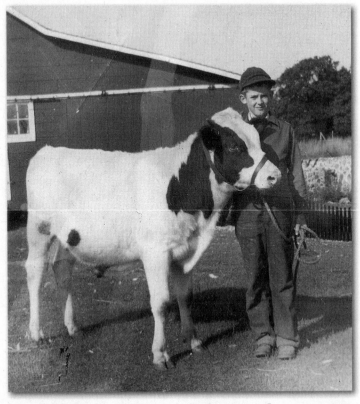

My 4-H calf, Stormy, and I learned a lot the summer I was recovering from polio. He had a mind of his own, as did I.

to show my calf at the county fair later that summer, I would have to teach him how to lead. Stormy, however, wanted nothing to do with halters and halter ropes and limping 4-H kids trying to teach him anything.

To get started each day, Pa would help me corral Stormy in the calf pen and put on his halter. He also helped me "lead" him outside—this consisted mostly of pulling and shoving and swatting Stormy on his behind to get him to move. The little bull enjoyed running around the barnyard without a halter, but once the halter was in place, he was the most stubborn creature that had ever set foot on our farm. He would shake his head with its little black horns back and forth and defiantly plant his front feet as if to say, "I dare you to make me move."

Once we got Stormy outside, I was on my own. Nearly every day, two things happened. First, Stormy refused to take one step. He stood like a black-and-white statue with what I came to believe was a smile on his face, his dark eyes glaring at me. I don't think they glared with hatred; I always believed the little bull liked me. He just didn't want anything to do with learning how to lead. The second thing Stormy would do, every single day but without warning, was to take off running with me holding on to the rope. Yelling "stop" made no difference—indeed, I believe it encouraged him. I wasn't strong enough to yank him to a stop with the halter rope, so I simply held on, usually falling down and dragging behind him across the yard. My bad leg prevented me from running to keep up, but my arms and shoulders grew stronger each day as I refused to let go of that rope. I had the cuts and scrapes and dirty bib overalls to show for my daily adventure.

Day after day it was the same thing: full stop, followed by out-of-control go. After a month of this I told Pa that I was ready to give up. Stormy was never going to learn how to lead. I said nothing about my gimpy leg keeping me from running after the little bull when he took off. I didn't want to offer an excuse. I merely wanted to make the case that this particular little bull calf would never learn how to lead.

As Pa listened patiently to my story, I thought I could see a hint of a smile on his face. Of course, he had been watching these goings-on each day, but he had made no comment and offered no advice for how I could convince this little Holstein that things would go better for everyone if he'd simply allow himself to be led around the yard with rope and halter.

Near tears, I finally declared, "I'm not going to do this anymore. My leg hurts, my arms are scraped and scratched, my hands are burned from the rope—and besides, Stormy doesn't wanna learn how to lead!"

All the while, Stormy stood there, looking at us, listening—and I'll bet understanding too. He had won the battle. No more daily aggravation from this limping 4-H member.

"So, you're giving up?" Pa said.

"I am. It's no use. He'll never learn to lead."

"You're sure?"

"I'm sure."

Pa didn't say anything for a time, which was his way. When there was a difficult moment, a decision to be made, a crisis to face, he often said nothing. If asked about his moments of quiet, he would say, "Sometimes it's best to let the dust settle before saying or doing anything." Clearly this was a "dust settling" moment.

So the three of us stood there on the grass between the house and the barn, the sun shining brightly down on us. Stormy was nibbling grass as I stood holding the halter rope. Finally, Pa said, "Hand me that rope."

Stormy lifted his head and looked at Pa, and Pa looked at Stormy.

"Let's go," Pa said. With Pa holding the rope, Stormy walked along next to him, doing everything my father asked him to do. Stop, turn, move faster, move slower: no problem at all. The little calf knew how to lead, no question about it. Pa walked as far as the granary, turned, and walked back to where I stood watching, dumbfounded.

Pa was smiling when he handed the halter rope to me. I think Stormy was smiling too. "You gotta let him know who's boss," Pa said.

I felt terrible. All the while I had thought Stormy was never going to lead, and he had already learned—he just didn't want me to know it. The problem was me. I was feeling sorry for myself once again. If I had two good legs, this wouldn't have happened. But I knew better than to say this to Pa. By this time I'd learned that Pa would not accept an excuse, no matter what it was. I stood there, dumbly holding the halter rope, with the little bull calf looking at me, no doubt wondering what would happen next.

"Okay, Stormy," I said. I stood up straight, straightened my cap, and took a firm hold on the halter rope. "Let's go."

I walked forward, and Stormy walked alongside me as he was supposed to do. Once or twice he threatened to bolt, but I gave a sharp tug on the halter rope and he continued walking at my pace.

"Looks like you taught him pretty good," Pa said. I didn't answer. "Next thing you'll want to work on is teaching him how to back up."

"What?" I said. "I just got him to go forward without running away."

"Backing up is a little harder to teach. Not a natural thing. Calves don't normally do a lot of backing up."

"So why do I have to teach him how to back up, then?"

"Couple of reasons. So you can back him out of his stall, and, for the short run, because the cattle judge at the county fair will ask you to back him."

"Oh," was all I could think to say.

After that day, Stormy and I got along much better. I got him to back a few times, but he didn't like doing it, and I wasn't at all sure he would do it when a cattle judge asked. He took off running a few times too, though I realized it was probably my fault because I wasn't holding the rope firmly enough and he sensed he could get away with something. When I worked with Stormy, there was no letting up. I had to be constantly alert and aware of what I was doing. There was no halfway in leading this smart little calf.

The summer days slid by in a hurry, early mornings helping with a few barn chores, the rest of the morning in church, studying to be a good Lutheran, whatever that meant. During the afternoons I helped with farm work. After the milking was done in the early afternoon and the cows were turned out to pasture, I worked with Stormy, improving his leading skills—which still required considerable honing.

Soon it was mid-August and time for the Waushara County Fair, held each year at the fairgrounds in Wautoma. Pa called Ross Caves, the area cattle trucker, and arranged for him to haul the Chain O' Lake 4-H animals to the fair. Ross charged a dollar per animal, round trip, which even in those days was right next to being a gift. Along with Stormy, Ross would transport calves to the fair for several of my fellow 4-H members: Kenny Owens, Jim and Dave Kolka, Jerry York, and Joyce Dudley. He would pick them up in his big red cattle truck that made weekly trips to the stockyards in Milwaukee, where he delivered veal calves, hogs, worn-out milk cows—whatever animals local farmers had for sale.

Caves and his cattle truck arrived at our farm on Thursday around noon. The calves had to be in place at the Wautoma fairgrounds by five o' clock, as the fair opened that evening for its four-day stand.

"Say, Jerry, you're doing pretty well," Caves said when he saw me. He had obviously heard about me having polio, and I guess he was surprised that I was walking around and getting ready to show a calf at the county fair.

"Can't run," I said. "Still limping."

"Lots of folks limp," Caves said. "Your pa said you're showing a bull calf. Bull calves can be quite a handful."

"Yes, they can," I agreed. I limped to the barn, slipped the halter on Stormy, and led him to the ramp that stuck out from the back of the truck. He walked right up the ramp and into the truck without missing a step. I handed Caves the halter rope so he could tie it to one of the metal rings fastened inside the truck.

"Nice bull calf you got, Jerry."

"Kind of stubborn," I said. Caves smiled.

I walked around to the front of the truck where I could see Stormy's nose poking between the wooden slats. I petted him on the head and noticed he was shivering. He was clearly afraid.

"I'll see you in a little while," I said as I rubbed his forehead. He liked having his head rubbed. I've often thought that farm animals have a sense of foreboding whenever they walk into a cattle truck—with good reason, since for many animals the ride in a truck would be their first and last ride, as the destination was usually the stockyards, and then the slaughterhouse.

Pa and I arrived at the fairgrounds just ahead of the cattle truck, so I could lead Stormy from the truck to his stall in the cattle barn. The barn was already about half full with 4-H calves from throughout the county. I found a stall in the area set aside for bull calves, tied Stormy to the manger, spread fresh straw under him for bedding, and pulled some alfalfa hay from a gunny bag we'd brought from the farm. He soon settled down and began eating hay, a good sign.

Pa left for home. I walked to the far south end of the fairgrounds, past the rides that would begin operating after five (a Tilt-a-Whirl, a merry-go-round, a Ferris wheel) and several games of chance (knock over the milk bottles, toss a wooden ring and win a watch). I passed a couple of hamburger stands, the smell of fried onions reminding me that it would soon be suppertime. Under a small stand of oak trees, not far from the fairground fence, I spotted the 4-H tent. It was a used tent, left over from World War II, but it seemed like a perfect place for the boys in our 4-H club to sleep so they would be handy to take care of their calves. Clayton Owens, our 4-H leader, had also bought several army surplus folding canvas cots. It would be my first time sleeping in a tent, and I thought our home away from home was as pleasant as pleasant could be. Kenny, Jerry, and the Kolka boys were already there. We talked about the fair, about the judging that would begin the next day, and about where we thought we could get a deal on something for supper. We decided that a short walk to downtown Wautoma would be best, thinking we could get more food for our money there than at the fairgrounds.

My only concern was whether I could walk the half mile or so to town—and even more troubling, whether I could keep up with my fellow 4-Hers. It was the sort of thing that bothered me a lot in those days, worrying that I would be unable to do what others could do without even thinking about it, and even worse worrying that I would cause others to do things—like walking more slowly—just because of me. I shouldn't have worried, as I was able to keep up with everyone with no difficulty. Soon we were on Main Street, and I could see the restaurant sign a half block away.

Families didn't eat out in restaurants much in those days, and I remember having done so only once or twice by that time. Now my 4-H buddies and I sat around a big table in Wautoma's Main Street Restaurant, staring at menus that the waitress had handed us. Not sure what to choose, we all decided to order the plate lunch, which included thick slabs of roast beef, a pile of mashed potatoes with brown gravy, and a healthy portion of green beans. The price was sixty-five cents, and for a nickel more we could have a bottle of Coca-Cola or Orange Crush. I ordered the Orange Crush, something I'd never had before. It was cold, sweet, and bubbly—and much more delicious than the canned orange juice I'd had to drink when I was sick. When my meal arrived, my appetite seemed to disappear, and I had some difficulty swallowing. But I managed to eat, not wanting to let my buddies know that I had a problem.

Despite my difficulty, it was a fine meal in every respect, and I didn't hear a single complaint from anybody in our group. I suspect that like me most of them had no experience in a restaurant, and I'm guessing the waitress quickly figured out that we were 4-H kids fresh off the farm and staying at the fair. I didn't look at what other customers were eating (Ma said you should never stare at other people), but I'm guessing the cook piled a couple of extra slabs of beef on our plates and more than the usual amount of mashed potatoes.

With our bellies full, we all walked slowly back to the fairgrounds, enjoying the coolness of the evening. We checked on our calves to make sure they were well bedded and fed, and then ambled across the fairgrounds toward our tent. By this time eager fair visitors had begun arriving. The rides were in full operation, the midway was alive with the sounds of the barkers trying to entice people to their little canvas-covered booths, and the smell of fried onions filled the air around the food tents. It was an exciting, noisy, crowded place. So different from life on the farm.

Clayton Owens said we'd better turn in early, as we had to be up by five thirty to prepare our calves for judging, which would begin at nine. With all the sounds and smells of the fair going on around us, I can't say we went to sleep promptly, but eventually we did.

Before six the next morning we were all in the cattle barn, feeding and watering our calves, cleaning up behind them, and hauling fresh bedding. The most important job of all was preparing our calves for the show ring. It was sort of like going on a first date—you wanted to look just right and make a good first impression (of course, at age twelve I knew nothing about first dates). If your calf looked clean and well brushed, you knew the judge would at least give the animal a decent score during the judging.

I brushed Stormy until his black-and-white coat shined. Next, I washed his flanks to remove any evidence of manure stains. Before coming to the fair, Pa and I had clipped the long hairs from his tail, leaving an ample brush at the end. We had clipped the long hairs on his head, too, so his big eyes seemed even bigger and his horns even larger. Pa had taught me to use black shoe polish on his horns, and they shone blacker than usual. Now I polished Stormy's halter with shoe polish, rubbing the leather until it shined.

I had Stormy ready by eight o'clock, leaving me an entire hour to wait and make sure that Stormy stayed clean—and to worry about how Stormy would act once I began leading him in a circle with other bull calves. Pa, Ma, and my little brothers arrived at the barn about eight thirty. Pa said that Stormy looked real good, and Ma told me she'd brought along a picnic lunch. My brothers said they wanted to go looking around, that they weren't much interested in cattle judging, but Pa told them no, they'd better watch, because in a few years they'd be showing their own 4-H calves at the fair.

I listened to the loudspeaker announcing which classes were about to be judged and soon heard, "Junior Holstein bull calves." This was it. I untied Stormy from his manger and led him outside, holding tight to the strap of the show halter that Pa had bought for me at Gorman's leather shop in Wild Rose. Pa walked alongside me. I'm sure he was as concerned as I was about Stormy's erratic behavior. Would the little bull decide he wanted no part of this and simply take off running, with me stumbling along behind? Or would he behave himself? I'd soon find out.

I spoke quietly to Stormy as we walked together into the show ring, where four or five other little Holstein bull calves and their handlers had already gathered. Some of the little bulls were acting up, jumping around and giving the boys leading them a challenge. But not Stormy; he walked beside me, behaving better than he ever had. The cattle judge, a county agricultural agent from a neighboring county, stood in the center of the show ring, which was surrounded with a four-foot-high wood-and-wire snow fence. The judge said nothing; he just stood there, looking at each bull calf as he and his handler came into the ring.

"This is it," I whispered to Stormy. The little bull seemed to understand as he walked with his head high, doing exactly what I asked of him. Together we walked around the ring twice, Stormy a perfect gentleman, unlike several of the other little bulls that continued to challenge their handlers.

After our second walk around, the judge motioned for me to lead Stormy to the center of the ring and stop. I was elated. Unless the judge changed his mind, Stormy would receive first place. When all the little bulls were lined up in rows from first place to fourth place, the judge went to each calf.

"Back your calf," the judge said to me.

I pulled on the show halter, and Stormy backed just like I had taught him. No complaint, no refusal. Perfect performance.

"Thank you," the judge said. "Lead him back into position, please." I did so without a misstep. The judge went down the line, asking each 4-H member to back his calf. Some of the calves complied; most of them didn't.

When I walked out of the show ring, I carried a blue ribbon in my hand and wore a big smile on my face. I think Stormy was smiling too. I don't know if little Holstein bulls can think, but I had the idea that Stormy was thinking, *We sure showed that judge, didn't we?*

Later that morning, all of the first-place calves were invited back into the show ring for the showmanship contest, in which both the calf and calf's handler were judged at the same time. Once more Stormy let everyone know that he knew how to lead, how to back, how to hold his head high, how to do everything I asked him to do, better than any other 4-H kid and his calf. The little bull calf and I won the showmanship contest.

Pa was about as proud as he could be. He didn't say much, no back patting or "You did good," but he did say, "Stormy's quite a calf. Quite a calf." He was smiling when he said it.

I hadn't felt this good in a long time. For a little while, thoughts of my bad leg faded into the background. I had done well, had even competed with kids who had two good legs, and I had won. But it had not come easy. I had spent many hours with Stormy, most of them troublesome, trying hours. As I look back now on my relationship with my little bull that summer, it reminds me of the time I spent with Pastor Renner and my confirmation lessons. At the time I could see little reason for learning (memorizing, really) tons of what I considered irrelevant stuff. I'm sure Stormy felt the same way about learning how to lead. I learned an important lesson that summer: no matter what might get in the way, hard work, patience, and perseverance can make a difference, even when the challenge seems impossible to overcome.

## 12    Wild Rose High

Labor Day was fast approaching, and with it the beginning of the fall term of school. This year I would not be walking with my brothers down the dusty country road to the one-room Chain O' Lake School, but climbing on a school bus for the four-and-a-half-mile ride to Wild Rose High School. It would be a new adventure, and I was scared out of my wits. I'd heard tales of what city kids did to country kids—hicks, as we were called. And I had three additional things working against me. I was young for my grade, having just turned thirteen in July. I was also small, not yet five feet tall. And worst of all, I limped and couldn't run without falling. My leg had gotten much stronger over the summer, but I couldn't avoid the limp. It had become a part of me.

In fall 1947, Wild Rose High School sent out its first school buses, two of them, painted red, white, and blue. Before that, country kids made their way to high school as best they could, walking, catching rides with friends, or even boarding in town. The high school principal, Wilford Engbretson, owned the buses; he drove one, and his farmhand drove the other. My folks paid $1.25 a week directly to the principal for the bus ride.

On the first day of school, I was surprised to discover that after picking me up, the bus did not transport me directly to the high school. No indeed. I climbed on the bus at 7:30 a.m., and we bounced all over God's creation for nearly an hour and a half. Principal Engbretson drove us two-thirds of the way to Plainfield, picking up kids along the way; from there he drove north of Wild Rose toward Waupaca, on dusty roads I'd never traveled, roads so rough I had to grab hold of the seat in front of me in order to stay put. We picked up more and more kids: little kids, big kids, kids I'd never seen before. We drove and drove and bounced and bounced, and I began to feel sick. Some of the other kids looked a little green as well. I sure was glad when the bus pulled up in front of the high school and the principal pulled on the door handle. We all staggered out.

When I got off the bus, Bob Zubeck stood waiting for me. Bob was a neighbor kid who had graduated from Chain O' Lake a year ahead of me. As a sophomore, I'm sure he wasn't too happy about following his mother's suggestion that he look after me on my first day of high school.

"Hi, Jerry," he said when he spotted me.

"Hi, Bob," I muttered. I was still getting my land legs after the long ride and felt a bit wobbly standing in front of the enormous school. The building housed an elementary school on the first floor and the high school on the second floor. Attached at the north side of the two-story main building was a one-story gymnasium built by Works Progress Administration workers during the Depression.

"We've got a few minutes before school starts, so I'll show you around," Bob offered. I followed along as we entered the big building, the smell of recently cleaned floors floating up around us. Kids were everywhere. I'd never seen so many kids in one building before. Our country school never had more than twenty-five or thirty students enrolled at one time. This school obviously had several times that many. I asked Bob how many kids attended the high school, and he said about a hundred. I thought, *that's sure a big bunch of kids to have on one floor of one building.*

Bob led me to the basement and showed me the boy's bathroom, which contained a short row of urinals, something I had never seen before, and several stalls of flush toilets, also something I'd had little experience with, as we had no indoor plumbing at home or at Chain O' Lake School. "Sure is a fancy place," I said. Bob didn't respond.

Then he took me upstairs to the second floor. He showed me where the principal's office was located. "That's a place where you never want to find yourself," he said. "You only go there when you're in trouble."

He pointed out the library, a sizable room containing more books than I had ever seen in one place. Books covered two walls from floor to ceiling, many times more books than were on the few bookshelves at my country school. I couldn't wait to do more exploring in this room—and I also figured I'd have to be selective, because I couldn't possibly read all these books in four years.

Finally, Bob dropped me off at the freshman homeroom. "See you around," he said. I was on my own.

I opened the door and saw my freshman classmates staring at me. I was the last one to enter the room, just barely on time. "You must be Jerry Apps," a balding older man at the front of the room said. He wore a brown suit with a necktie. "I'm Mr. Wright, your homeroom teacher. Find an empty seat." He smiled.

That year Wild Rose High School had ninety-seven students in all four grades. My freshman class included six girls and eleven boys, one of the smallest freshman classes in the years before and after. Six teachers composed the faculty: Wilford Engbretson (principal, introductory science, introductory mathematics); Arlene Holt (English I, II, III, IV, and librarian); Mae Songe (typing, shorthand, social science); Alden De Shetler (music); Helen Wieczorek (biology, home economics); and Paul Wright (algebra, geometry, US history, world history, speech, basketball coach, baseball coach—there was no football or track at Wild Rose High).

I looked around the room and saw but one familiar face, Kenny Owens from my 4-H club. He smiled at me, and I smiled back. I didn't think I'd seen any of the other kids before. About half of them were town kids. The rest came from several country school districts that sent their eighth grade graduates to Wild Rose High. I wondered if any of the other kids were as scared as I was.

As I sat through my first freshman math class, I found that it wasn't too difficult. Most of what Mr. Engbretson was teaching I knew from my grade school arithmetic class. I went on to freshman English and met Miss Holt, and then to Mrs. Songe's social science class. While we were preparing to leave for lunch, an older kid came up to me. He was a good head taller than I was but was kind of pale and skinny. I took him to be a town kid. "Do you know how to hand wrestle?" he asked. He spoke with a kind of snarl.

"No, I don't," I answered, not sure what he wanted me to do.

"Oh, it's easy," he said. He held up his hands with fingers spread. I couldn't see any calluses on his hands.

"What we do is, we put our fingers together and try to bend the other guy's hands back—try to make him kneel."

I thought this seemed like a dumb kind of wrestling, but I agreed to it. When we had our hands laced together, the boy said, "On the count of three, start pushing." He had kind of a mean smile on his face.

"Three!" he suddenly said. He began squeezing my fingers and pushing my hands back, bending my wrists.

He had taken me by surprise with his phony count, but as soon as he began squeezing and pushing, I squeezed and pushed back. Before you could say, "Let's try this again," he was kneeling and saying, "Stop, stop!" I let go. As he got back to his feet, I noticed he had tears in his eyes. What that kid didn't know was I milked cows by hand every day, and my fingers had more strength than even I was aware of. He never asked me to hand wrestle again. If only my bad leg was as strong as my hands.

Wild Rose High School did not yet have a lunchroom, and the school lunch program was set up in the basement of the Masonic Hall on Main Street in Wild Rose. The elementary kids walked over and ate first, and then starting at 11:30 the various high school classes walked the several blocks to the back door of the Masonic Hall and down the steps to the basement. There we stood in line to pay twenty-five cents and receive a ticket for lunch. What I remember most about the lunch was how poorly the green beans tasted compared to those we had on our home farm. Of course, the beans we ate at home were fresh; we ate them only an hour or so after we picked them. The green beans in the school lunch program sat around in big cans for weeks, maybe months. I remember the school lunch hot dogs being quite tasty, on the other hand; we almost never had them at home, so they were a treat. I ate the school lunch every day that week, until my mother decided she could pack me a sack lunch for less than twenty-five cents a day. (On top of the $1.25 a week for bus fare, the lunch expense was probably more than my folks wanted to invest in my high school education.) I didn't tell my mother this, but I also felt uncomfortable eating with a group of kids. With a sack lunch, I didn't have to sit at a table with a bunch of other kids but could crawl off in a corner someplace and eat by myself.

That afternoon I found my way to geography and general science classes. This was the first time I had experienced different teachers teaching different subjects. I knew this would take some getting used to—no more sitting in one room with one teacher all day. That first day of high school I tried to do what my dad always said he did whenever he faced a new situation: "First you've got to learn the lay of the land." I continued to follow that advice for the next several weeks at school. I kept my eyes and ears wide open and didn't say much, only answering when I was asked something. But that didn't mean I wasn't aware of what was going on around me.

As he was showing me around the school that morning, Bob Zubeck had suggested I try out for the baseball team, which he'd called one of the best in the league. "Every freshman boy tries out for the team," he told me. "It's the thing to do." I had promised him I would—even though I had never played baseball in my life. Softball was my thing. But I didn't want to say no and immediately be cast as an outsider at my new school.

In those days the school mascot was a wild rose, and the teams were called the Rosies, a title that I'm sure put fear and trepidation in their opponents (today Wild Rose High's teams are known as the Wildcats). Baseball tryouts were held after classes got out that afternoon. The baseball diamond was located just east of the high school, on a spot of ground that had no trees, quite unlike our softball diamond at Chain O' Lake. The pitcher's mound even appeared to be a bit higher than the rest of the bases, which were stuffed pieces of canvas about a foot square—real bases. Home plate was a piece of board painted white, five-sided and lying flat against the ground.

The older team members helped Coach Wright with tryouts; Cliff Simonson, a junior, was the team's pitcher, and Marty Inda, also a junior, was catcher. They were a formidable pair. Cliff had a pitch that would set even the most seasoned player back on his haunches when he fired off an inside fastball. And Marty—well, I never saw him drop a pitched ball, and could he ever throw to second base to catch a potential base stealer. Of course, I didn't know any of this my first day of high school when I was waiting in line to take my swings at the plate, scared to death.

Coach Wright lined up all the freshman boys who wanted to try out for the team: Dave Jones, Alan Walters, Kenny Owens, Eddie Schmidt, and me, the shortest kid on the field. Dave had been attending the town elementary school, and it was clear that he knew baseball as he walked up to the plate, took a couple of practice swings, and hit the first pitch well past second base.

"Okay, Apps, it's your turn," said Coach Wright.

I limped up to the plate. "Stand a little closer," said the coach. I edged a couple inches closer. Marty Inda was kneeling just behind me, his face covered with the metal catcher's screen, his chest protected with pads.

Bob Zubeck had told me to hold the bat off my shoulder, and so I did. I looked out at Cliff Simonson standing high up on the pitcher's mound, pounding the baseball into his glove. Once, twice. Whap, Whap. Then he went into his windup. I could feel sweat on my forehead. I held tight to the bat.

I saw the ball coming—coming fast, and straight for my head. It was Cliff's famous inside fastball, I later learned. The next thing I knew, I was on the ground and looking up at a circle of people looking down at me.

"Are you all right?" Coach Wright asked. "Are you all right?" I felt my head where the ball had hit me. A huge lump had appeared.

"I...I don't know," I stammered. Cliff Simonson helped me to my feet, looking concerned. "Never hit a kid in the head before," he muttered. "Never did."

I didn't say anything. Several kids and Coach Wright helped me to a bench, where I sat down, still dazed from the fastball that had knocked me out for a few minutes. I knew what had happened: my gimpy leg hadn't moved fast enough for me to get out of the way. I knew right then and there that I wouldn't be playing baseball for Wild Rose High. In fact, my experience at tryouts that day foretold my involvement in sports throughout my high school years: nil. I couldn't move fast enough for either baseball or basketball.

That evening when I climbed off the bus at the end of our driveway, I left my books on the kitchen table, changed my clothes, and headed out to the barn for the evening chores. My mother wasn't in the house; she was probably working in the garden.

"Well, how'd it go?" Pa asked when he saw me. He was scattering cow feed in the mangers before letting in the cows for the evening milking.

"Okay," I said, as I began helping him. He didn't push me for more. I didn't tell him about being knocked out by a baseball—he didn't need to know about that. I also didn't tell him how terrible I felt, not just because my head was now aching from that pitched ball, but because I was unable to do what the other freshman boys could do, play baseball. I felt about as low as person could feel. I surely wasn't looking forward to four years of high school and being the one constantly left out. I was glad none of the other kids had made fun of my inability to get out of the way of Cliff's fastball. Maybe Coach Wright had said something to them—I never found out. Nonetheless, I wasn't looking forward to the next day of school, or to four years of feeling worthless.

# 13　*The Rose-Bud*

By the time I was a sophomore at Wild Rose High School, I was outwardly confident and self-assured—and inwardly a mess. I was president of the sophomore class, a member of the student council, on the academic honor roll, and announcing the basketball games. But most days I felt about as worthless as anybody could feel. My recuperation from polio had stalled. I could walk, even run a little, but I continued to limp. Sometime I tripped, when my right leg didn't want to keep up with my left. And I would never be able to play high school basketball or baseball, which nearly all the boys in my class could do.

I had become afflicted by something else too, something that would take me many years to overcome. I could not eat comfortably away from home and in front of other people. The problem had started after my illness and had gotten steadily worse. When I look back on it, I think this surely was a manifestation of feeling worthless. Of course, my folks rarely took us out to a restaurant. But I discovered that even eating at a relative's home, something my family did fairly often, was a challenge. My folks noticed this and took me to see both Dr. Hadden and another Wild Rose doctor, Dr. Hong. Both were general practitioners, and neither thought I had a medical problem beyond the lingering physical effects of polio. Using different words, they said the same thing: it was all in my head. They were right, of course.

During my freshman and sophomore years, I carried a bag lunch to school, which I could eat comfortably with a friend or two during lunch. By the time I was a junior, one of the teachers asked if I would like to sell school lunch tickets. In return I would receive a free lunch, but I would have to eat early, a little after eleven. I would be able to eat in the cafeteria, which by this time was in the basement of the high school. At that early hour, no one was around except the cooks, so eating was not a problem. And my mother would no longer have to pack a lunch for me each day.

It had nothing to do with having had polio, but by my sophomore year my handwriting had gone from bad to worse. That year I enrolled in a typewriting class, which in those days was a part of what was called the "commercial major"—meaning that after courses in typewriting, shorthand, and business methods, you could find a job in an office someplace. It was an attractive option for many of the high school girls in those days. I had no intention of working as a secretary, but I did know that I was interested in writing. And if I wanted anyone to be able to read what I'd written, I had better learn how to type.

In the second semester of my sophomore year, I sat in the typewriting room, a big L. C. Smith manual typewriter parked in front of me and rows of girls sitting around me, all with similar typewriters. I was the lone boy in the room. I looked around at the girls in the class, all of whom seemed to have long, skinny fingers.

I figured that these were the kind of fingers typewriter makers had in mind when they designed the machines. I had short, thick fingers, calloused from farm work. They were tough, scarred, and strong from my thumb to my little pinky, nothing dainty about them. I immediately thought that typewriting was going to be a challenge for my clunky farmer hands.

I had never once worked a typewriter. Everything about the machine was new to me. What I quickly learned was that a manual typewriter required strong fingers. To type on a manual typewriter, you had to poke at each key with considerable vigor, or nothing much happened. I discovered that my fingers worked just fine on a type-writer keyboard—better than most of the girls, who as it turned out had weak pinkies. When you're using the touch-typing method—and that was the only kind of typing allowed in class (no hunt and peck)—the pinkies are required to strike the *a* on the left and the *;* on the right. There isn't much call for semicolons, so the right pinky is mostly off the hook. But not so for the left pinky. Lots of words have an *a* in them.

Before we could do anything else, our typing teacher, Mrs. Schaeffner, insisted that we memorize the keyboard so that we could type in the dark if necessary. If she caught us looking at the keyboard while typing, we were in trouble. Once I had memorized the home keys for the left hand (*a, s, d, f,* and *g*) and for the right (*j, k, l, ;,* and *'*), I was on my way to learning the entire QWERTY (or as I thought of it, "quirky") keyboard layout.

Years later I learned that Christopher Latham Sholes, a Wisconsin newspaperman, had patented the first practical "Type Writing Machine" in 1868. It was Sholes who discovered that if the typewriter keys were organized in alphabetical order, they would quickly jam. He organized the keys in an efficient order based on their frequency of use: the QWERTY format—a keyboard design we use to this day, and which I am using as I type these words (without looking at my fingers, I might add). In 1873 Sholes sold the rights to the Remington Arms company, which began manufacturing Remington Typewriters in 1874. During my sophomore year, I spent some hard-earned money for a Remington Rand portable typewriter, a machine that I still have, although it's been years since I used it.

Once we had memorized the keyboard, Mrs. Schaeffner directed us to type, over and over, "The quick brown fox jumps over the lazy dog." I thought it was about the dumbest sentence I'd ever typed, until it dawned on me that it contains every letter of the alphabet, all twenty-six of them. Quite clever, really.

Typewriting class became one of my favorites. It took next to no thinking, especially compared to such classes as algebra or geometry. I enjoyed the feeling of the keys under my fingers, the neat appearance of letters all in a row on the paper in front of me, the sound of the keys striking the paper, and the ding of the little bell telling me I was at the end of a line and needed to throw the carriage and start a new line.

After a few weeks, Mrs. Schaeffner began giving timed typing tests once a week. Before you could say, "That kid milks cows by hand," I was winning the typing competitions. Soon I had earned a little forty-words-per-minute pin. To my surprise, I had discovered a physical thing that I could do better than other kids. My right leg didn't work very well, by my fingers were just fine—better than fine.

I also learned that the high school newspaper, called the *Purple and Gold* then, was closely tied to the typewriting class. The students on the newspaper staff wrote the news stories, but members of the typewriting class typed them in their final formats for the paper. A local printer printed the newspaper, which was nine by twelve inches and just four sheets long. With ads on the fourth page and most of the third, the paper essentially contained only two pages of news, both high school and grade school events.

In the fall of 1949, my junior year, the school newspaper made two major changes. The name became *The Rose-Bud,* and the newspaper staff began printing the newspaper on a recently purchased spirit duplicator, located in the typewriting room. The first edition in 1949 consisted of twelve pages, with two pages devoted to ads. Unfortunately, the print quality was considerably uneven—the type was a kind of bluish purple, with some letters dark and readable but others so light they were barely visible. But now the students were in charge. In October 1949 I became the advertising manager for *The Rose-Bud,* which meant I helped hustle ads for the paper. In November I was promoted to assistant editor, probably because I was the world's worst ad salesman, but I'd become a better than average typist. I quickly discovered that the editor and the assistant editor not only wrote most of the articles but also helped type them as well.

One thing I prided myself in doing as I moved along in my high school newspaper career was spotting dumb jokes in magazines and other newspapers and stealing them for *The Rose-Bud:*

*"Your husband has a new suit."*
*"No he doesn't."*
*"Well, something's different."*
*"It's a new husband."*

*What did the skunk say when the wind changed?*
*"It all comes back to me now."*

*The teacher was testing the knowledge of the kinder-garten class. Slapping a half dollar on the desk, she asked sharply, "What is that?"*

*Instantly a voice from the rear of the room said, "Tails."*

I also sprinkled in "words of wisdom" found in such magazines as *Reader's Digest* and farm papers:

*"It is better to be alone than in bad company."*—George Washington

*"I will prepare and someday my chance will come."*—Abraham Lincoln

*If you think you'll lose, you've lost,*
*For out in the world you'll find*
*Success begins with a person's will—*
*It's all in the state of mind.*
*Life's battles don't always go*
*To the stronger or faster man;*
*But sooner or later, the person who wins*
*Is the fellow who thinks he can.*—Anon.

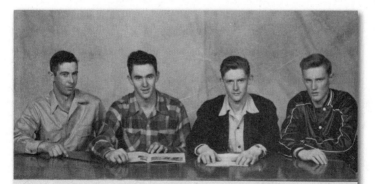

## ANNUAL STAFF

Editor . . . . . . . . . . . . . . . David Jones
Assistant Editor . . . . . . . Roger Gertenrich
Circulation Manager . . . . . . Douglas Jenks
Advertising Manager . . . . . . . Jerold Apps
Advisor . . . . . . . . . . . . . . Miss Holt

Seated:  C. Towne, D. Jones, J. Kolka, J. Apps, P. Etheridge, A. Walters, Mr. Harvey.
Standing: V. Huber, I. Chase, D. Jenks, D. Fenrich, D. Simon, J. Zubeck, B. Nelson, A. Peterson.

## NEWSPAPER STAFF

I served on both high school annual staff and newspaper staff, seen here in 1950.

# The Rose-Bud

February 1951.

## Washington

He made Our Country Free,

## Lincoln;

He kept Our Country Free.

Somebody did a golden deed,
  Somebody proved a friend in need
Somebody sang a beautiful song
  Somebody smiled the whole day long;
Somebody thought "Tis sweet to live"
  Somebody said "I'm glad to give",
Somebody fought a valiant fight,
  Somebody lived to shield the right,
Was that "Somebody You?"

Wild-Rose High-School.          Auth.unknown.

The front page of *The Rose-Bud* for February 1951. I liked to say the paper included "All the news that was fit to print—and more."

In the fall of 1950, when I was a senior, I became editor of *The Rose-Bud* and supervised a staff of twelve responsible for putting out a monthly newspaper. What fun it was. I did much of the writing: news stories, "food for thought," history pieces, and even news from the country schools that fed their students into Wild Rose High. My little brother Donald was the reporter for my old country school, Chain O' Lake. Among other things, he wrote, "Our civics class has been learning to be good citizens and have learned what it costs our parents to maintain a school."

Of everything I wrote for the newspaper, the editorials were the most fun to do. I could write just about anything I wanted—my editorials had to pass muster with the newspaper advisor, Bill Harvey, and with Mr. Ruzicka, by this time the school's principal, but I never had a problem with censorship. I wrote about Lincoln and Washington, spring fever, and the history of Santa Claus. In the Christmas editorial for December 1950, six months after the start of the Korean War, I wrote, "Everyone realizes the terrible crises the world is now experiencing. We are again engaged in war, which may lead to World War III. More now than ever before we should work for peace on earth good will toward men."

My time working on *The Rose-Bud* confirmed my interest in writing, enhanced my confidence about my ability to write, and probably most importantly, provided me with a special something I could do well, bad leg or no. Everybody at Wild Rose High looked up to the sports stars, those who excelled in baseball and basketball. But everyone also read *The Rose-Bud,* and they let me know what they liked and didn't like in no uncertain terms. What else could a writer hope for?

# 14  Mr. Wright

One thing I realize as I look back at my high school years is that there were people along the way who understood my difficulties and were looking out for me. One of those people was Paul Wright, Wild Rose High's baseball and basketball coach and the teacher of many subjects. Mr. Wright was in his early sixties, bald, round faced, always smiling, and a bit overweight, though he probably had been very athletic as a young man, and he was a great coach. At the time he seemed an unlikely person to care about a skinny little limping kid from the country who didn't smile much and looked like he didn't have a nickel in his pocket. But he did worry about me, more than I realized at the time.

During my sophomore year, I took algebra with Mr. Wright; I liked the subject, and it came easy to me. Mr. Wright was the sophomore class advisor, so I also saw him outside of algebra class. One day he suggested that I help some of my classmates who were struggling with this foreign form of mathematics. I worked with students during study halls and at noon, and I liked doing it. I quickly discovered that by helping others I increased my knowledge of the subject as well. That fall my classmates elected me class president. *What an undeserved honor,* I thought. I couldn't even play baseball or basketball.

When basketball season began that winter, Mr. Wright asked me if I would consider being the announcer for some of the home games. I asked him what I'd have to do. "Oh, you just sit up in the bleachers with the microphone, and when a player does something important, you announce it."

Ordinarily I was as shy as a farm boy could be. But with that microphone in my hand, everything changed. Occasionally one of my classmates sitting near me at a game told me to shut up, since they all could see very well who was making a basket and they didn't much care how many points he had accumulated. I replied—with a bit of microphone-induced arrogance, I must confess—that some of the folks in the audience *didn't* know who was who, and it was my job to let them know. Besides, folks needed to know that my classmate Allen Walters was a really good basketball player (he was also one of those who was having a dickens of a time with algebra, but of course I didn't let the world know about that).

That September, I received a scholarship to attend a 4-H conservation camp held each year at Camp Anokijig, near Little Elkhart Lake in Sheboygan County. I was the only Wild Rose High School student to go. The experience would cement my lifelong interest in nature and the environment.

Camp Anokijig's stated purpose was "to enlarge our lives by increasing our interest and understanding of the things of nature about us, and to learn that stewardship of natural resources is a citizen's first responsibility." From the start of the camp on a Wednesday to its close the following Saturday, I learned about glaciers and the

Kettle Moraine, went on nature hikes every morning, learned about geology in a lime pit, got my feet wet in a trout stream, hiked through a marsh, and visited a virgin hardwood forest. I learned about tree planting and heard lectures about how wild animals fit into the environment and the importance of soil conservation. I didn't know at the time that some of the top experts in these fields from the University of Wisconsin, the state conservation department, and other state agencies were our speakers and tour leaders. I even had the chance to meet Wakelin McNeel, whom I knew as Ranger Mac. I had listened to many of his *Afield with Ranger Mac* radio programs, which were broadcast to country schools throughout the state as a part of the Wisconsin School of the Air.

After a full day of activities, each evening we sat by the shores of the lake, around a blazing campfire, and recalled what we had done that day and what it had meant to us. It was a wonderful several days. On the last day of the camp, we all recited together the national conservation pledge: "I give my pledge as an American to save and faithfully to defend from waste the natural resources of my country—its soils and minerals, its forests, waters and wildlife."

Sometime during my first winter of sports announcing (perhaps thinking of some of the offhand comments I made at one of the games), Mr. Wright told me I had a reasonably good speaking voice but that I needed to polish my delivery. To do so, he encouraged me to participate in the interschool public speaking program called forensics. I had eight years of public speaking experience at Chain O' Lake School, especially in the annual Christmas program, when each student had to stand up and say his or her piece, plus perform in skits. But those were only short pieces, nothing like what we were supposed to do in the forensics program.

That winter and spring I practiced speaking along with the other students in the forensics program. Mr. Wright gave us tips that ranged from how to breathe to how to project our voices, from how to look at the audience to how to effectively use notes when speaking.

By my senior year, Mr. Wright encouraged me to try the original oration emphasis in forensics, meaning I would write my own speeches rather than memorize something someone else had written. It occurred to me that I could tie together my interests in the environment and nature, writing, and speaking. Original orations proved far more challenging, and more interesting too, than any other part of the forensics program. Writing

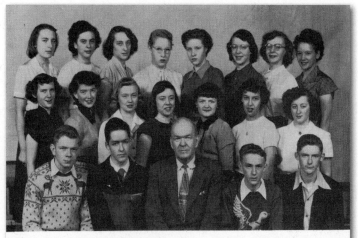

Row 1: N. Bryen, L. Eserhut, Mr. Wright, J. Kolka, J. Apps.
Row 2: D. Walters, R. McKnight, A. Peterson, K. Keohane, K. Colligan, N. Towne, R. Nowland.
Row 3: J. George, M. Swendrzynski, V. Huber, A. Korleski, J. Bartleson, A. Brownlow, I. Chase, G. Hirst.

# FORENSICS

Wild Rose High School Forensics Club, 1950–1951. I am at the far right.

an original oration required researching the topic, then writing and revising the piece, and finally delivering it to an audience.

I decided to combine my interests in nature and writing by preparing a conservation speech, which I titled "The Hole in Uncle Sam's Pocket." I labored over the speech, writing and rewriting it several times. Mr. Wright read each draft and offered suggestions for improvement. Although he didn't teach English, he nonetheless was a stickler for proper English, both written and spoken.

I still have the original copy of that speech, now more than sixty years old, wrinkled and yellowed. In it I wrote, "The conservation needs of our country are at the most critical point they have ever been in the history of our nation. Everyone can and must practice conservation of our natural resources if our nation is to retain the superiority we have had in the past." Though I wrote that in 1950, I could write it today and it would be as timely as it was then.

That winter I won the regional forensics event in Almond. From there I would head to the district event in Stevens Point, where I would compete against original speechwriters from all over central Wisconsin. As bad luck would have it, I came down with pneumonia a week before the Stevens Point event. I crawled out of bed to participate at the district competition; my voice was weak and my stamina nil. But I made it through the speech, which had been my goal. I took second place.

Since writing "The Hole in Uncle Sam's Pocket," I have written and delivered more than a thousand speeches, and I'm still doing it. I know now how much Mr. Wright's encouragement helped improve the speech

THE HOLE IN UNCLE SAM'S POCKET

What boy has not lost some of his treasures thru that forgotten hole in his trousers pocket? Important as these losses were however, they were soon forgotten in the excitement of new events and experiences. Uncle Sam, however, is allowing treasure to trickle thru a hole in his pocket, and he knows the hole is there! Some small repairs have been undertaken but so far the golden stream has been only slightly retarded. Of course you know by now to what I refer. The leak I mean, is that terrific loss of natural resources due to neglect, carelessness and down-right waste.

Methods for curbing these losses are referred to under the general title of conservation. This field of conservation is much to large to be covered in a short speech so I will touch on only three phases of it.

Every year, the farms of the United States lose three billion tons of top soil by erosion. This loss, figured in dollars, would represent a figure close to a third of a billion. This soil, if formed into a foot square column, would reach six hundred times around the world.

For the 1950 high school forensics competition, I wrote and delivered an original oration titled "The Hole in Uncle Sam's Pocket" about the importance of soil conservation.

and my delivery of it. At a time when I considered myself a loser and believed I was destined to always be one, Mr. Wright's support largely kept me going. Had he said but one discouraging word, I would have given up speechwriting on the spot.

It was Mr. Wright's influence again that got me involved in drama. I hadn't been in a play since country school, and there the plays could best be called skits. But at Wild Rose High the senior class was responsible for putting on a full-blown school play, performing it for the entire community. In addition to all his other responsibilities, Mr. Wright directed the school plays.

I don't remember there being tryouts for the various parts. By this time we had but fifteen students in our senior class, four girls and eleven boys, and Mr. Wright knew each of us quite well. He simply decided what parts each student would play. There wasn't any, "I'd rather do this," or, "I don't want to do that." We all had too much respect for Mr. Wright to question his decisions.

The title of the play was *The Patsy: A Three-Act Comedy.* I played the role of Bill Harrington, and Joan Nordahl was Mrs. William Harrington, my wife. I had never had to memorize so many lines in my life; it was worse than memorizing the stuff from Luther's Small Catechism. But there was a major difference between the catechism and *The Patsy:* the play was a comedy. It was fun to work on a line until you said it just right, so that someone in the audience would at least giggle, maybe even laugh out loud.

The play had only nine roles, but nobody was left out. Everyone had a job to do. The kids who weren't

### Production Staff

| | |
|---|---|
| Business Manager | Donald Van Airsdale |
| Stage Manager | Allen Walters |
| Prompter | Kenneth Owens |
| Ticket Seller | Erwin Pone |
| Ticket Taker | Edward Schmidt |
| Make-up | Mr. and Mrs. O. Nelson |
| Junior Ushers | Jean Wilson and Kathy Keohane |
| Director | Paul H. Wright |

*Entertainment between acts by Donna Walters, Kathy Keohane and Jean Wilson*

Produced by special arrangement with Samuel French

### Cast of Characters

| | |
|---|---|
| Bill Harrington | Jerry Apps |
| Mrs. William Harrington | Joan Nordahl |
| Grace Harrington | Carol Towne |
| Patricia Harrington | Patty Etheridge |
| Billy Caldwald | Dave Jones |
| Tony Anderson | Dean Fenwick |
| Sadie Buchanan | Barbara Radloff |
| Francis Patrick O'Flaherty | Douglas Jenks |
| "Trip" Busty | Jerry Stewart |

### Synopsis of Scenes

ACT I
*Living room of the Harrington home. Evening.*

ACT II
*Same. Next Monday evening.*

ACT III
*Same. The Friday night following*

What fun it was to be an actor—for one school play. I had the lead in *The Patsy.*

picked as actors did everything from ticket taking to business and stage management. By this time I had a driver's license, and Pa let me drive the Plymouth to town once a week for play practice. He gave me strict instructions to drive no farther than to town and back—no running off to Wautoma for a root beer at the A&W drive-in. Even with all the memorizing, which I discovered wasn't all that difficult, play practice was great fun. Again I had found something I could do as well as—even better than—some of my classmates who had excelled in baseball and basketball. As I moved around the stage according to Director Wright's instructions, nobody noticed or seemed to care that I had a slight limp.

At the end-of-year awards program that spring, where basketball and baseball players received their school letter—a big gold W with a purple border—I received one too. Instead of a little gold basketball or baseball, pinned to my W was a gold lamp, signifying forensics. I couldn't have been prouder. Now I could wear a W on my high school sweater, just like so many of my friends.

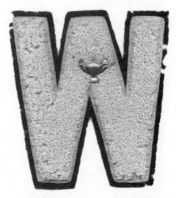

I was never more proud than when I received my W for forensics at the same time my classmates were receiving Ws for various sports.

Mr. Wright wrote something in each of our yearbooks at graduation time. He always wrote his comments in verse. In my 1951 yearbook, he wrote:

*Dear Jerry,*
*A few folks one can ne'er forget*
*And you are one now, you just bet.*
*And as through life our path does wind*
*Remember me as a good friend.*
*And e'er my rhyming instinct stops*
*I want to state I think you're tops.*
*But being a sorry fact, I fear*
*You won't be back another year.*
*Best of luck, Jerry.*
*Paul*

I suspect Mr. Wright wrote something similar in everyone's yearbook, but nonetheless I prized his comments then, and I still do. He was someone who made a difference in my life, a tremendous difference. He was there to help me when I needed help the most.

# 15   Good News

In early May 1951, as the end of my senior year was drawing near, Principal Ruzicka called me to his office. In my
four years of high school I had never seen the inside of
the principal's office—which I considered a good thing,
since those who were summoned there had usually gotten into trouble. Miss Holt, the school librarian, smiled
at me as I walked past her desk and reluctantly knocked
on the dreaded door to the principal's office.

"Come in," I heard. I entered, looking around at the
shelves of books and papers stacked here and there and
the file cabinets against the wall.

"Have a chair, Jerry," Mr. Ruzicka said. He had gray
hair and wore wire-rimmed glasses and a three-piece
suit and tie. He had a pleasant tone of voice, but others
who had been in his office said he usually started out a
conversation pleasantly. Then he got down to business,
and you learned why you were sitting across the desk
from him.

I didn't say anything; I was waiting for the other shoe
to drop. Was it something I'd written in *The Rose-Bud?*
Something he didn't like in the gossip column or in one
of my editorials? A complaint he'd gotten from some-

one? As a writer I'd quickly learned that you can't please everyone, and you shouldn't even try.

The pleasant voice continued. "Jerry, I've got some good news for you."

I still didn't speak, though I was taken a bit off guard. Good news is not what I was expecting to hear.

"The senior class advisor and I have been calculating the class rank," Mr. Ruzicka began. I didn't say anything. My mind was still in the "I must have been doing something wrong, and he's taking a long way around to tell me" mode.

He smiled and said, "You are the valedictorian of the senior class."

"What?" was all I could mumble.

"You are the top student in your class, Jerry."

I sat for a moment, allowing the news to sink in. Part of me wanted to say that he was wrong, that they must have made an error in their figuring.

"I am?" I said. Mr. Ruzicka laughed.

I knew I had been getting good grades and had been on the honor roll every term, but other students were on the honor roll as well. In those days, the goal was to do as well as you could in school. My folks had drummed into me the importance of working hard. "It's a great opportunity to go to school," they often said. But class rank was something I had never thought about.

"Douglas Jenks will be salutatorian," Mr. Ruzicka added. "Second place."

"Doug is a good student," I said. Doug was my friend. Indeed, with such a small class, I considered all fourteen of my classmates my friends. We worked together on many projects, often doubling up on jobs for big projects such as the senior class play and the senior dance.

We all got along well. I quickly wondered if receiving the nod as top student in my class would ruin some of these friendships.

"I have other good news for you too," Mr. Ruzicka said. Again he paused and smiled. "As valedictorian you will receive a semester's free tuition to attend the University of Wisconsin in Madison."

I couldn't believe what I was hearing. I had given little thought to going to college. Few students went to college then; high school was considered a major achievement. And I knew my family had little money to pay for extra education, so I had pushed the idea of college from my mind. I hoped to stay on the farm and work alongside my dad. But I also knew that with my bum leg, farming would be a challenge.

"We've got to let the UW know in a week or so whether you'll accept the scholarship."

"I'll talk to my folks," I said.

I left Mr. Ruzicka's office with my head in a whirl. I had expected a chewing out for something or other, and instead I learned that I had the top grades in my high school class. To think that I'd also receive a scholarship to the University of Wisconsin! I had been to Madison once, on a 4-H field trip when we visited the capitol. I had never been to the UW campus. And I wasn't at all sure what my folks would think about me going to college.

As the school bus bounced along the country roads that afternoon, dropping off students here and there, I was deep in thought. For four years I had felt sorry for myself because I couldn't play basketball, baseball, or track, which had been added recently at Wild Rose High. In order to compensate, I had studied hard, read widely, done all my assignments, written quite a bit, and helped

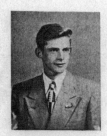

**JEROLD W. APPS**
"Judicious, Willing, Ambitious"
Newspaper 3,4; President 2,4; Forensics 4; Student Council 2,4; Annual Staff 4; Newspaper 3; Newspaper Editor 4; Treasurer 3; Baseball 1; Volleyball 1,2,3; Badger Boy State Award 3; Class Play 4.

**DAVID R. JONES**
"Daring, Risky, Jolly"
Basketball 1,2,3,4; Baseball 1,2,3,4; Track 3; Volleyball 1,2,3,4; Newspaper 3,4; President 1; Treasurer 2; Vice President 3,4; Student Council 1; President Student Council 4; Annual Staff 3,4; Annual Editor 4; Homecoming King 3; Class Play 4.

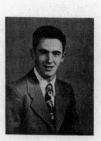

# SENIORS

President . . . . . . . . . . . . . Jerold Apps

Vice President . . . . . . . . . . David Jones

Secretary . . . . . . . . . . . Patty Etheridge

Treasurer . . . . . . . . . . . Douglas Jenks

Student Council . . . . . . . . . . Erwin Pone

Advisor . . . . . . . . . . . . . . Miss Holt

Class Flower . . . . . . . . . . . Yellow Rose

Class Colors . . . . . . . . Scarlet and Silver

Class Motto . . . . . . . . "One step at a time
and always forward"

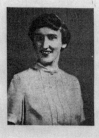

**PATRICIA L. ETHERIDGE**
"Playful, Likeable, Eloquent"
FHA 2; Skating Club 2,3,4; Newspaper 3,4; Cheerleader 3,4; Forensics 3; Basketball 1,2,3,4; Prom Queen 3; Homecoming Court of Honor 3,4; Glee Club 2,4; Mixed Chorus 4; Treasurer 1; Secretary 2,3,4; Flag Twirling 4; Class Play 4; D. A. R. Award.

**DOUGLAS A. JENKS**
"Devilish, Able, Joyful"
Student Council 2,3; Newspaper 4; President 3; Treasurer 4; Volleyball 1,2,3; Annual Staff 4; Class play 4.

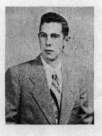

Here I am pictured in our 1951 Wild Rose High School Annual, along with my fellow senior classmates. I hold the record for the shortest career in high school baseball, one pitch that hit me in the head. I also stumbled along through volleyball as part of the required physical education program.

my fellow students when they asked. I had gained some self-respect with my writing and public speaking successes, but I had a long way to go. I still wanted to do what the other guys in my class did: compete in sports. I saw the fun they had with their teammates, and I envied that they could travel around the area playing other schools. I had many friends in my class and in other grades—thanks in part to my work on *The Rose-Bud*. But I also spent a lot of my time by myself, reading, writing, walking in the woods, doing solitary things. I was fine with that; I didn't need to have others around me all the time. I was slowly learning to live with myself, and perhaps more importantly I was beginning to accept and appreciate what I could do well instead of dwelling on what I could not do and would never be able to do: compete in athletics and other activities that required two good legs.

Pa often said, "Do the best you can with what you've got." I suspect I didn't appreciate those words at the time I first heard them, but they have stayed with me my entire life. Nowhere in Pa's words was there an implication that you should try to better someone else, to compete with them. There's nothing wrong with competition, I suspect, but it can lead to envy and jealousy. Better to worry about competing with yourself, doing something better than the last time you did it. Pa also said, "It doesn't much matter what you do, there is always someone who can do it better and someone who can't do it as well." What he was saying was, keep your eye on where you're headed, and spend less time looking around at those ahead of you and those behind you.

At the same time, my pa had high standards, and he believed in having something to strive for. He would conclude this discussion with, "Keep an eye on those who do something especially well, no matter if it's how to take care of cows, how to plow in a straight line, or how to figure in your head." Years later one of my professors at the university would add another twist to this line of thought. He said, "Good enough is never good enough." Those words had great meaning for me. Doing something well enough to get by is not acceptable, for ultimately it leads to mediocrity.

When I arrived home that afternoon, I changed my clothes, asked my mother what was for supper, and went out to the barn where Pa was doing the early evening chores. He was carrying in oat straw for the calf pen from remnants of the straw stack that in the fall had stood tall alongside the west side of the barn. I grabbed a fork to help.

When we'd finished bedding the calves, I said, "Pa, I learned something today in school."

"Well, I hope so," he said, smiling.

"I mean, I learned something beyond the regular stuff."

Pa leaned on his fork handle and looked at me.

"I'm going to be valedictorian of my high school class. Mr. Ruzicka told me this afternoon," I said. I tried to keep any excitement out of my voice, which was plenty hard to do.

"Well, that's good," Pa said.

"There's something else."

Pa continued looking at me, puzzled as to what I was going to say. Having never attended high school, everything I was telling him was new.

"I also will receive a scholarship for one semester's tuition at the University of Wisconsin in Madison. If I want it," I quickly added.

For a long time Pa said nothing. He had kind of a sad look on his face, not the look of excitement that I had hoped for. I had an idea what he was thinking. As the oldest son, I knew he was expecting me to stay on the farm. He had watched me work the last few summers and had seen the strength of my leg improve to the point that I could do almost all farmwork without difficulty, as long as I didn't have to do any running.

After what seemed like forever, he asked, "How much is that university scholarship worth?"

"Sixty-three dollars and fifty cents," I said. "Enough to cover my first-semester tuition."

He thought again for a time, though less time than before.

"That's a lot of money. You'd probably better take them up on the offer." Then almost as an afterthought, he asked, "What do you want to take up at the university?"

"I was thinking about studying agriculture, maybe becoming a high school agriculture teacher."

"That's good. You might learn something we could use here on the farm."

We continued doing the barn chores without saying a word. That evening at the supper table I told Ma my good news, and she seemed happy about it, but I could also see questions etched on her face.

"How in the world are we gonna scrape up enough money to send you off to college?" she wondered aloud. "Since we had to sell those cows, we scarcely have enough money to make ends meet."

Earlier that year, several of our best milk cows had tested positive for brucellosis and by law had to be destroyed. With our best cows gone, Pa had bought some very ordinary milk cows so we would have some income. But they didn't hold a candle to the production of our Holsteins. We'd have to wait for the heifer calves to grow up before the herd would return to some semblance of what it had been before brucellosis showed up on the farm.

"They're offering me a scholarship for the tuition," I said.

"Still, you've got to eat," Ma replied. "You need a roof over your head. And you can't run around the university campus wearing patched bib overalls and a straw hat." I smiled at her reference to the clothing I wore around the farm during the summer. I was more worried about limping my way around campus than about what other college kids might have to say about what I was wearing.

"We'll try and figure something out," Pa said quietly. "We could plant a bigger pickle patch—still some money in growing cucumbers. Got room for a bigger green bean patch too. Beans are still selling pretty good. We'll all have to work a little harder."

I was dumbfounded to find Pa squarely in my corner. Ma's reaction didn't surprise me. She was the bookkeeper in the family and knew exactly how much money was coming in and how much was going out. And I could see from the looks on my brothers' faces that they weren't too keen on bigger cucumber and bean patches, because they would be picking them along with the rest of the family. But with Pa's backing, the decision was made. I would be the first one in the family to attend college.

My dad's support for my going to college was a turning point in my life, for had he said I should stay on the farm, I would have done so. Later I overhead one of my uncles tell my dad that the only reason a boy goes off to college is to get out of work. Pa simply didn't respond.

When I returned to school the following day, I told Mr. Ruzicka that I would accept the scholarship and that I looked forward to attending the university in the fall. He said he was pleased with my decision. I didn't tell him about the conversation we'd had at home, and how Ma especially was concerned about how the family would afford the cost of college.

At our high school graduation ceremony I sat on the stage along with Mr. Ruzicka and the president of the school board. As valedictorian, I was to give a short speech. I don't remember much of what I said, other than expressing how humbling it was to represent the Class of 1951 as both class president and valedictorian. Pa's words were in my head: "Whatever you do, don't brag. Nobody likes a bragger. Let your actions speak for you."

I had only fifteen minutes to speak, and the time sped by. I could see my folks in the audience, looking as proud as I had ever seen them. My brothers were there too, along with some of our neighbors. And then the ceremony was over. Back at home Ma took my picture wearing my graduation gown and standing in front of one of her flower beds. There was no graduation party, just a special meal Ma fixed that evening. After supper, with the rented graduation gown safely back in its box, I pulled on my

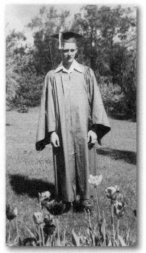

In 1951 high school graduation was an important day; for many students it meant the end of their formal schooling.

bib overalls and accompanied Pa to the barn for the evening milking.

As I worked, my head was a swirl of thoughts about the past four years. I had discovered that even though there were some things I would never be able to do, I could excel at other things, such as writing and speaking. My high school years had also reinforced my love for learning, discovering new ideas, and realizing that I had the freedom to think my own thoughts and write and speak about them. Above all, I was beginning to come to grips with the aftereffects of polio, both its physical and psychological manifestations.

The cucumbers and beans grew well that summer, and the harvest was above average. Nobody talked about it much, but we all knew that the entire family was pitching in so that I could go to college.

I completed the application for admission to the University of Wisconsin's College of Agriculture and in a couple of weeks learned that I had been accepted. Along with the admission materials, the UW sent information about the dormitories on campus. Ma and I studied the costs for the dorms, including the meal plans. She finally said, "We just can't afford having you stay in a dorm."

I didn't say anything. I knew nothing about dorm life at a university. But when I envisioned a bunch of kids all staying in the same building, I wasn't too keen on the idea. Even at age sixteen I enjoyed and appreciated solitude. It was when I was alone that I did my best thinking, my best studying, and my best writing.

In August Ma and I went to Madison to look for a place for me to live. Not long before, Pa had traded the 1936 Plymouth, which was on its last legs, for a used 1950 Chevrolet. I'd gotten my driver's license the previous summer, so I was at the wheel when we headed for Madison on that warm August day. In my admission materials I'd found the address for the University Housing Office, on Sterling Court at the east end of the campus.

After a long two hours of driving, we arrived at the outskirts of Madison and stopped at a gas station for directions. "Where is Sterling Court?" I asked the gas station attendant.

"Never heard of it."

"It's near the UW campus," I said.

"Still never heard of it."

We drove on, stopping a couple of times for directions but with the same results. When we finally found Sterling Court, we discovered it was just one block long, which was probably why nobody knew about it. Ma and I walked up the steps and into the housing office. We spotted a bulletin board with a long list of rooming houses and their prices. We saw a listing for a second-floor room at 112 North Orchard Street. Ma asked the person at the desk where that might be. The woman pointed in the general direction and said, "Drive down University Avenue, and when you come to a big hospital on your right—that would be University Hospital—turn left onto Orchard Street."

We found the address with no difficulty. It was a big, old three-story house, one of many we drove past on and around the campus. Soon we were talking to Mr. and Mrs. Roy Pein, the owners of the house. Ma explained that I would be attending the university in the fall and needed a room. Mr. Pein showed us the room they had for rent, a nice big room facing northwest. There was a sink in one corner. *What luxury,* I thought, *to have a sink right in your own room.* At home we did not yet have indoor plumbing.

The furnishings were modest: a bed, a dresser, a

rather beat-up study desk, a well-worn carpet on the floor, and a single light bulb hanging from the ceiling. It looked good to me.

"What's your rental rate?" Ma asked. She wasted little time in getting down to the important items on her agenda.

"Five dollars a week," said Mr. Pein.

"That a firm price?" Ma asked.

"It is," said Mr. Pein.

"Then I believe we'll take it."

"I'll need a check for twenty dollars to cover the first month." said Mr. Pein.

Ma dug into her purse, found the checkbook from the Union State Bank in Wild Rose, and wrote a check for twenty dollars. She tore it out, but not before filling out the stub with the appropriate information. She handed it to Mr. Pein and said, "Thank you."

"Thank *you*," he said.

Ma was pleased with my room. On the drive home she said that she knew where she could buy a used electric hot plate so I could cook some of my meals in my room. She had already observed where the electric outlets were located. "Be a lot less expensive than eating meals in one of those dorm cafeterias," she said.

I wasn't looking forward to living in the city, but my new room, where I would be all by myself, seemed like a good place. Besides, I still had a few weeks to get used to the idea that I would be a university student and a farm boy well out of his element.

# 16   New Student Week

With the whole family busy with barn chores, hay making, potato hoeing, grain harvesting, threshing, and cucumber and bean picking, the rest of the summer flew by. Through it all my bad leg seemed to work pretty well—about as well as it was ever going to work, I later learned. I fell into bed exhausted every night, only to start working again at 5:30 the next morning. I thought little about my upcoming studies at the University of Wisconsin.

By that summer of 1951, the Korean War was raging, and the draft was picking off young people one after the other. I wouldn't have to register for the draft until I was eighteen, more than a year off. But all of my high school classmates were at least a year older than me, and I knew they were worried about being drafted.

Soon it was September and only a couple weeks until the start of the fall semester at the UW. According to my admission materials, I was to attend New Student Week, September 17 through 22, before classes began on September 24. The week before I left for Madison, we filled our silo with green corn stalks, hard but satisfying work. The green corn bundles, cut with our tractor-pulled corn binder, were heavy but smelled wonderful. So many smells on the farm are distinctive: fresh-cut hay, newly threshed oats, the pungent smell of soil turned over while hoeing, the smells of a summer morning when dew hangs on everything and the sun just begins to creep over the horizon in the east, the tangy smell of corn silage beginning to ferment. I couldn't help thinking about how much I would miss those smells when I traipsed off to the university in a few days.

Pa would not drive in a city the size of Madison, so my uncle Wilbur Witt agreed to drive my mother and me to campus on Sunday, September 16. I gathered up my things and packed them into Uncle Wilbur's trunk: a new RCA Victor battery/electric-powered portable radio that I had gotten for my birthday, my Remington portable typewriter, fifty sheets of typing paper, a new ballpoint pen, two newly sharpened lead pencils, two new pairs of khaki pants (Ma thought these would look so much better than blue jeans), three new shirts, a rain jacket, and some new underwear. Ma sent along with me a sturdy mailing box that I was instructed to use for mailing my dirty clothes home each week so she could wash them— another way to save on expenses. I also had a brand new checkbook from the Union State Bank in Wild Rose, with a balance of $150. This money—a combination of my earnings from picking cucumbers and beans that summer and money contributed by my family—was meant to cover the purchase of my books and my meals for the first semester.

There was little conversation on the drive to Madison. Ma and I were both deep in thought. Uncle Wilbur was content to check the field crops along the way and the quality of the dairy cattle he saw grazing in the pastures. When we stopped at a little restaurant on the east side of Madison for lunch, my difficulty eating in a crowd returned in a fury. I could eat only a few bites of what I had ordered, much to the unhappiness of my mother, who didn't like to waste food and always worried when I didn't eat.

When we arrived at 112 North Orchard, Uncle Wilbur and Ma helped carry my meager possessions up to my room. It took only one trip with everyone carrying something. Uncle Wilbur told me good luck and shook my hand. Ma stood there for a minute, looking at me, and then she turned and left with my uncle. Our family was never much for hugging or kissing. I knew Ma was as concerned about my welfare as I was, but she didn't say anything. She didn't have to. I could see how she felt written all over her face. I could see it in her eyes.

I hung my new shirts and pants in my closet, placed my typewriter on the desk, unpacked my paper and pencils and ballpoint pen, and then sprawled out on my bed. It was midafternoon, and the sounds of the city filtered through the open window—unfamiliar sounds of cars and trucks and buses, horns blowing, even a siren wailing. I was accustomed to the quiet lowing of a cow on pasture, the subtle sound of wind caressing shoulder-high corn, the boom of thunder when a rainstorm boiled up in the west, the call of a whip-poor-will on a warm summer night. These were my sounds, the sounds I knew and understood. Would I ever come to know these city sounds as my own?

I paged through the instructions the UW had mailed me. I was to appear at the Fieldhouse at eight the following morning for the "official welcome." I wondered where the Fieldhouse was. When Ma and I had driven to Madison to find a room, we hadn't stayed long enough to look around the campus. I suspect Ma figured we wouldn't have enough time to do that and still be back home in time for the evening chores. So aside from the housing office, I had no idea where any of the campus buildings were. The place was a mystery to me.

Having eaten almost nothing for lunch, by five o'clock I was starving. (Luckily my problem with eating in a crowd diminished the hungrier I got.) I limped my way up to University Avenue, looked left, and saw a sign for a Rennebohm Drug Store. I knew they must have a lunch counter. I sat on a stool at the counter and ordered a hamburger with tomato and lettuce, plus a glass of chocolate milk, total bill: forty-nine cents. I would soon learn that Rennebohm's offered several items at forty-nine cents; in fact, they called their noon special a forty-niner.

While I was eating, I asked the waitress the location of the Fieldhouse.

"You're a new freshman," she said.

"Yup, I am," I answered proudly. It was beginning to sink in that I indeed was now a university student.

The young lady smiled. "When you go out the door, turn left and walk a couple blocks to Breese Terrace. Turn left on Breese and walk a few more blocks. You'll soon come to the football stadium, and on the south end of the football stadium you'll see the Fieldhouse. It's a big stone building."

"Thank you," I said. I finished my hamburger and decided that since I had nothing else to do, I would try to find the Fieldhouse now. Then I wouldn't have to worry about being late for the welcome ceremony on Monday morning.

By 1951 the University of Wisconsin was on the tail end of a great influx of veterans who had returned from World

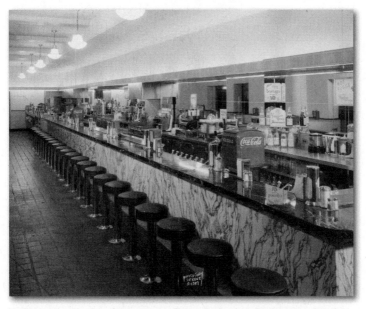

I often ate at the lunch counter at Rennebohm's, which was only a few blocks from my rooming house. *WHi Image ID 3979*

War II and received G.I. Bill benefits to attend college. In 1943 the UW student population had numbered just under six thousand, but by 1947 there were well more than eighteen thousand students enrolled. To accommodate the surge of students, the university had hurriedly built twenty-seven single-story temporary buildings of various sizes to serve as classrooms, office space, and even a cafeteria (at the corner of Breese Terrace and University Avenue). The temporary buildings included two Quonset huts, one north of the chemical engineering building and one north of the education building. I walked past several of these temporary buildings on my way to the Fieldhouse, which I found with no difficulty. From there I decided to walk a different route to my rooming house. I had always had a good sense of direction, and soon I was back in my room at 112 North Orchard. I wasn't accustomed to this much walking, and my bad leg reminded me of the fact. It tired much more quickly than my good leg, and I limped more noticeably when I walked a lot. I was glad to be back to my room for the night.

The next morning I was up at 5:30, my usual time for getting up, although for the first morning for as long I could remember, there were no cows to fetch from the pasture and no morning chores to do. The house was quiet as I used the shared bath, which had a bath tub and no shower. I wondered where I might find breakfast. By 6:30 I was on my way toward Rennebohm's again; the counter was filled with breakfast folks, none of whom looked like students. I ordered a big sweet roll, a glass of milk, and a glass of orange juice that came from a big container with a revolving paddle to keep it mixed. After my good supper the night before I had set a goal to never pay more than seventy-five cents for any meal. Breakfast was thirty-nine cents, if I recall correctly.

At 7:30 I stood at the door of the Fieldhouse marked New Student Week, waiting for it to open. Since Pa had been drumming into me my entire life that I should never be late for anything, sometimes I arrived a bit too early. Eventually the door opened, and I saw for the first time the inside of this enormous building. In the center was a basketball court, now covered with chairs, and surrounding that were bleachers all around, all the way to the ceiling. I couldn't help but stare. Later I learned that the Fieldhouse seated twelve thousand people. Most of the population at that time of my home county of Waushara could have fit in this one building.

I found a seat near the front where I could easily see the podium. Soon a sea of freshmen students, more than two thousand of them, were seated around me. I knew not one of them. A woman whose name I don't remember walked to the podium and addressed the crowd. She welcomed us to the University of Wisconsin and said we would all have an enjoyable experience, especially if we applied ourselves. "We are privileged to have with us this morning, for a few brief words of introduction, the president of the University of Wisconsin, Doctor E. B. Fred," the woman said. A round-faced, bald gentleman approached the podium, and everyone clapped loudly. I didn't know why. I had never heard of the guy, and besides, he hadn't yet said a word.

Dr. Fred's brief comments were far from brief and not especially interesting. Still, I tried to pay attention and not let my mind wander to all the other things I faced during this week of orientation to "the great University of Wisconsin," as President Fred described the place. I was quickly realizing that I'd better get used to calling these university bigwigs "doctor," even though I doubted any of them knew the first thing about curing a sore throat or telling me how to take care of my bum leg.

President Fred droned on about the University of Wisconsin's history, going back to 1848, the year Wisconsin became a state. "The first class," he said, "had only seventeen students, and they began meeting in February of 1849." He described how the UW became a land-grant university not long after President Lincoln signed the Morrill Act in 1862, making federal lands available to support public universities in each state. He explained that land-grant universities must have as a part of their curriculum studies in engineering, agriculture, and military tactics. "Of course," he said, smiling, "other courses of study are not excluded."

President Fred told us about a plaque bolted to the wall to the left of the main entrance to Bascom Hall (I had no idea where to find Bascom Hall) and recited the words inscribed there:

> *Whatever may be the limitations which trammel inquiry elsewhere, we believe that the great state University of Wisconsin should ever encourage that continual and fearless sifting and winnowing by which alone the truth can be found.*

He concluded by telling us that our years at the university would give us the tools, background, and perspective to carry out what was described on that plaque and to become thoughtful citizens of the world.

While the words meant little to me at the time, the idea of "fearless sifting and winnowing in the search for truth" has become a powerful mantra in both my professional and personal life. But as a college freshman, I was far too worried about doing well in my classes, figuring out how to live in a city, having enough money to stay in school, and limping around the huge campus to consider the meaning of those words.

My next New Student Week activity took me to Bascom Hall, perched on top of a hill in the center of campus with a view of the state capitol to the east. As I walked past a coppery-green statue of Abraham Lincoln seated in a big chair, I smiled to myself, remembering having overhead someone at the orientation session saying they'd heard that if a virgin walked in front of Lincoln's

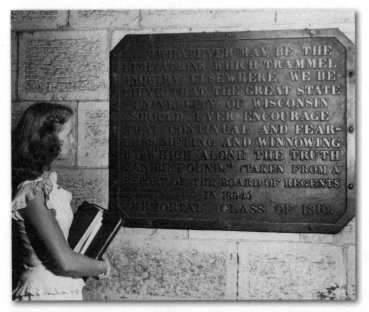

The "sifting and winnowing" statement on the plaque near the main entrance of Bascom Hall is as powerful to me today as when I first heard it in 1951. *WHi Image ID 57400*

statue, he would stand up. Reaching the front door of Bascom Hall, I glanced to the left and saw the plaque President Fred had spoken about. I stopped to read it, its deeper meaning still a considerable mystery to me.

I spent the rest of the day in Bascom Hall, seated in a huge room in a little wooden chair with a fold-up writing stand on the right side. There I took test after test—math, science, English, some kind of nonsense test with questions like "Apples are to oranges as railroad locomotives are to: _____." I had three choices to put in the blank: trains, highways, or airplanes. There were other tests too, all of them multiple choice. I hated multiple choice tests— I still do. I usually had more to say about a question than I could show by checking off a couple-word response.

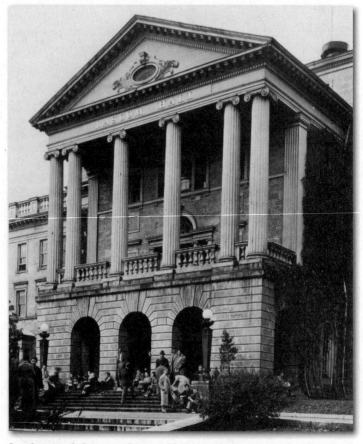

I took several classes in Bascom Hall, the administrative headquarters for the University of Wisconsin–Madison. *WHi Image ID 57222*

I returned to my little room on Orchard Street exhausted. My leg hurt from all the walking, and I had a fierce headache from sitting in a stuffy room all afternoon. I knew I had answered many of the test questions incorrectly. It had not been a good day.

The next morning at 7:45 I was scheduled to take a swimming examination in the pool at the Red Gym on Langdon Street—a considerable hike from my rooming house on Orchard Street, I discovered when I consulted my map. If you flunked the swimming test, you had to take swimming lessons until you passed. I had never been much of a swimmer—I could dog paddle some and had never learned to float—and I hadn't been swimming since I'd gotten polio because I just didn't feel comfortable doing it with a bad leg. And I had never in my life gone swimming in a pool.

I was in for one more shock (my first week at the UW was filled with them). We were instructed to shower in the locker room and appear at the pool buck naked. And so we did, no swimming trunks, no nothing, just a bunch of bare-assed boys staring off into space to avoid looking at each other, but sneaking a peak every so often to check on each other's physical attributes. We sat lined up all around the twenty-by-sixty-foot pool, the instructor at one end, also naked as a jaybird. It was a sight to see. In my furtive glances I noticed a few farmer tans like mine, but not many. I thought about what would happen if a girl stumbled upon us. Would she ever be in for a surprise! It wasn't until much later that I learned the reasons for the nude swimming rule. In 1951 polio was still on everyone's mind. To prevent the spread of the disease, swimmers in the Red Gym pool showered with strong soap and jumped into the pool unclad to make sure no germs made it into the pool water, which was brought to the pool from nearby Lake Mendota. A second reason had to do with plumbing: residue from the cotton swimsuits of the time would plug the pool's sand-and-gravel filtration system.

To begin the test, three of us at a time swam the length of the pool for a few laps using any stroke we chose. I dog paddled, and that part I passed. Doing more than one swimming stroke—that part I flunked. Next we were told to tread water for three minutes. After a minute or so, my bad leg gave up on me, and I was embarrassed when the instructor pushed a long pole in my direction and hauled me out of the pool. Thankfully, I wasn't the only one to flunk the swimming test. But I was now destined to take swimming lessons three times a week until I could pass it. And so I did, all that fall, hating the feeling of jumping into a swimming pool naked, feeling the treated water stinging my eyes. But not only did I pass the swimming test later that fall, swimming turned out to be great therapy for my leg.

The next day I learned what Army Reserve Officers Training Corps—everyone called it "Rot-C"—was all about. The UW required two years of ROTC training for all male students; two additional years were optional. Seated in another huge lecture hall, I listened to an army officer who talked like a machine gun telling us that if we stayed on for all four years of ROTC, we could become second lieutenants in the infantry, corps of engineers, signal corps, military police corps, or transportation corps. Next I listened to an air science officer talking about the air corps. He said that if we completed four years of ROTC training, not only could we become second lieutenants, we might be eligible for jet pilot training. I immediately decided to enroll in air science ROTC.

The military representatives reminded us of something we were well aware of as young men in 1951: the country was in the midst of the Korean War. Then they told us something I hadn't known: as long as we were enrolled in ROTC, we had draft deferments. It was an interesting situation, I thought: join the army to get out of it—or at least, to postpone serving. I probably could have avoided both the draft and ROTC duty by mentioning that I had had polio and had a less-than-perfect right leg and knee, but I mentioned this to no one.

On that same Wednesday of New Student Week, all freshmen enrolled in the College of Agriculture met in the Agriculture Hall auditorium for our official welcome to the college. In the course of my orientation that week, I had learned that the university included both schools and colleges—the college of letters and science, the college of engineering, and the college of agriculture; a school of home economics, medical school, school of nursing, school of education, school of commerce, school of pharmacy, and law school. Somehow to me it seemed more prestigious to be enrolled in a college than a school.

As I limped up the many steps to the Agriculture Hall entrance, I noticed that long ago someone hadn't known how to spell *agriculture*. The word carved into the masonry above the door read *Agricvltvre*. I found my way to the auditorium—more steps—and selected a seat near the front. Before long about 125 of us were seated there: the freshman class for 1951–1952 in the ag school, as we soon began calling it. Among us were only three girls. (In the 1951–1952 school year there were 608 students enrolled in the College of Agriculture; only eight of them were women.)

Dean Kivlin, associate dean for the College of Agriculture, walked onto the stage and took his place behind the podium. "Welcome to the College of Agriculture," he began. He told us that the university had a long and proud record of groundbreaking research in agriculture, from Stephen Babcock's invention of the Babcock milk tester to nutrition studies that resulted in the discovery of several vitamins. In fact, the first agriculture courses had been taught there in 1851, well before Wisconsin

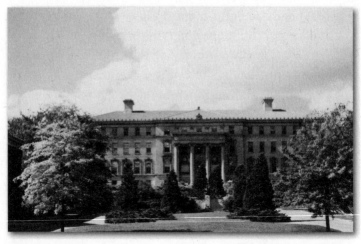

Many of my classes were held in Agriculture Hall. *WHi Image ID 55506*

became a dairy state. Although I found this history more interesting than Dr. Fred's speech of the day before, at the moment I had more basic questions on my mind. I wanted to know what courses I had to take to become a high school agriculture teacher. I quickly decided I wasn't going to learn much about that in this session, but I tried to look interested nonetheless. Then Dean Kivlin said something that nearly jarred me out of my chair.

"Look to your left and to your right," he said. We all did as he said, a little confused. "One of you will not be here in the spring."

That was not something I wanted to hear. I had enough misgivings already about this place, and now a highfalutin dean was telling us that a bunch of us wouldn't make it through the first semester. These comments surely didn't increase my optimism about attending college.

On Thursday I was scheduled to meet with my academic advisor, Dr. Bucholtz, who had offices in Moore Hall on the ag campus. That morning while I was eating my now-standard breakfast at Rennebohm's, I asked the waitress if she knew the whereabouts of Moore Hall. She said she'd never heard of it. The fellow sitting next to me at the counter, overhearing me, said he had never heard of that building either.

I started walking toward Agriculture Hall and met an older gentleman carrying a briefcase. I made him out to be some kind of professor; at least, he looked like other professors I'd met that week. I asked him if he knew where I might find Moore Hall. He smiled. "Sure. Walk just past Ag Engineering, and there you'll spot it on the left. Most of us call it the Agronomy Building." I headed off in the direction he'd pointed. Finally, I would learn what courses I must take.

Moore Hall was a fine old brick building, larger than any I'd seen in all of Waushara County. It was maybe twice as large as the Wild Rose Mercantile, the largest building in my home town. It was also two buildings in one. Attached to one end, forming an L, was the Horticulture Building. Of course, both agronomy and horticulture are about growing things, although at the time I didn't understand the nuanced differences between the two areas of study.

I pulled open the big front door of the Agronomy Building and walked down the hall until I found Professor Bucholtz's office. I still didn't know if I was supposed to address a college teacher as "Professor," "Dr.," or "Mr." Pa always told me, "It doesn't make much difference if the guy is a doctor, a lawyer, or some other high-up mucky-muck, he still pulls on his pants one leg at a time." I decided on "professor."

I quickly discovered that Professor Bucholtz was just an ordinary, nice guy—friendly, too, as he shook my hand

and asked where I was from. After a bit of chitchat about the kind of farming we did back in Waushara County, my new advisor took out a pad of paper and began writing down the required courses for freshmen in the College of Agriculture. "The first two years are mostly required courses, essentially the same ones that everyone takes," he told me. "The final two years are when you work on your major."

Two required noncredit courses—physical education and ROTC—headed the list, taking up six hours of class time a week. The credit courses Professor Bucholtz scratched on the notepad in front of me were:

Chemistry 1a, 5 credits

Animal Husbandry 1 (Livestock Production), 3 credits

Agronomy 1 (Principles and Practices in Crop Production), 3 credits

English 1a, 3 credits

Agriculture Engineering 5, 3 credits

Total, 17 credits

Hours in class or laboratory, 24

By the time he'd finished listing the required courses, I had room for just one elective that semester. I selected an agriculture engineering course. I told Professor Bucholtz about my plans to become a high school agriculture teacher. He said I'd probably want to change advisors for the spring semester, but that he'd help me get started this fall.

I left his office clutching the list, pleased to finally have an idea of what I'd be doing all semester. But I discovered that registering for my classes wasn't anywhere near as simple as it had been at Wild Rose High. I spent much of that day running around campus, looking for buildings and assignment committees (for courses with high enrollment), where my name was added to others in laboratory sessions, quiz sessions, and discussion sessions for my ROTC, English, and chemistry courses. When I'd completed the assignment committee business, thankfully not necessary for my agriculture courses, where the enrollments weren't so high, I found myself standing in a long line at the stock pavilion on the agriculture campus, where several people looked over my papers, stamped one of them, and declared me registered. But I wasn't quite finished with the process. I still had to walk all the way back to the east end of the campus, to a place called the Bursar's Office, where I was supposed to pay my tuition money. I told someone at the Stock Pavilion that I had a scholarship that covered my tuition, but he said I had to appear at the Bursar's Office nonetheless.

By this time in the registration process I had done a *lot* of walking, and my bad leg was aching. I climbed up Bascom Hill again, traversing its hundreds (well, maybe not that many) steps on the west side and then down the long, steep sidewalk on the east side. Once more I stood in a long line, this one leading to a clerk's window that looked a lot like the ones at the Union State Bank in Wild Rose, with a shelf at waist level and a window above the shelf where you could shove through a check. When it was finally my turn, a pleasant woman asked my name. I told her and explained that I had a scholarship that was supposed to cover my tuition for the fall semester.

She scanned through several sheets of papers and then looked up. "Yes, you do—but you still owe us $11.50, which includes the student fees." Apparently my scholarship wouldn't cover the entire seventy-five-dollar tuition after all. I wrote a check for the balance and handed it to her. She stamped yet another paper, smiled again, and that was it. I was now a student at the University of Wisconsin, bad leg and all.

Next I stopped at the University Co-op Bookstore and explored the shelves there to find the books required for my courses. I wrote another check, this one for fifteen dollars, and then hobbled back to my Orchard Street room and collapsed on my bed with mixed feelings. On the one hand I felt pretty good about being a college student, but on the other I wondered if I would be able to adjust to a place with thousands of students and buildings scattered all along Lake Mendota. I was uncertain whether I could do all the walking necessary to get from one class to another, when the classes were not down the hall like in Wild Rose High, but maybe a half mile away on the other end of campus. And I wondered how I would adjust to living in a city. The city noises—sirens and trucks—still woke me up at night. They were such harsh sounds, not at all like the quiet, subtle sounds of the country. I wondered if I would ever adjust to them, and part of me thought, *why should I adjust?* These were the sounds of urban living, and I was a country person. I would never be comfortable in the city—at least, that's what I thought at the time.

While I was already missing my life back on the farm, I vowed then and there never to tell anyone that I had grown up without electricity, that I had lived in a house heated by a woodstove and with no indoor plumbing, and that my early education had been in a one-room school-house. I wasn't ashamed of my upbringing, exactly, but I decided to keep the details of my background to myself. I wanted people to think that I was a cosmopolitan person who knew the ways of the world.

I also decided never to mention my experience with polio. When a student who lived at my rooming house saw me walking down the sidewalk and said to me, "You walk just like you are walking behind a plow," I replied that I had been doing just that not long before. I didn't tell him that part of the reason for my limp was having had polio. I immediately started watching how city people walked, and I worked on improving my walk so I could mostly pass for a city person. But I soon discovered that living in the city and attending a big university would require more of an adjustment than merely learning to "walk city."

# 17  First Semester

On Monday morning I was off to my first class, swimming at the Red Gym. From there I had to walk all the way across campus to the dairy barn for my animal science class. What a way to start the morning: a cold dip in the pool followed by a fast walk—as fast as I could, anyway—to make it to the dairy barn in fifteen minutes. At least the smells in the dairy barn were familiar ones, and I relaxed a little as I listened to Professor Grummer lecture us on the care and management of hogs, something I already knew something about.

My next class was chemistry lecture in the chemistry building on University Avenue. I found myself in a lecture hall larger than the movie theater in Wautoma. Nearly every seat was occupied by the time I got there; I guessed at least two hundred eager, and some not so eager, freshman students sat waiting for the professor to appear on the stage at the front of the auditorium. We each had a little folding table at the side of our seats, the same type I had become acquainted with in Bascom Hall a few days earlier.

Promptly at 8:50 the professor, a tall, thin, intense man, appeared on the stage in front of the room. "Good morning," he said, "and welcome to Chemistry 1a." I didn't know if I should say good morning back or just sit with my notebook and pen at the ready. I just sat.

"You've all had chemistry in high school," he began, "so much of the first six weeks will be mostly a review of what you already know." I relaxed a little. I had indeed taken chemistry in high school. The professor began writing on the blackboard, half turned toward all of us, talking nonstop. Before he'd gotten fifteen minutes into his lecture, I was lost. I took notes furiously, copying what he had scratched on the huge blackboard behind him, but I had no idea what I was writing. I didn't even recognize most of the words he used. My chemistry teacher at Wild Rose High hadn't used these words . . . at least, I didn't think he had. I began to wonder if over the summer I had forgotten a lot of what I should know. At the end of class I left the lecture hall worried.

I soon discovered that chemistry was only one of my worries. My next class was English 1a, which I had really been looking forward to. I wanted to improve my writing skills, and an English class is where I believed it would happen. The English class was a much smaller group, perhaps only thirty students. I felt a bit more comfortable, but not for long. The professor, a big, burly man with a shock of black hair and a deep voice, strode into the room, turned to the class, and without so much as a hi, hello, or good morning, launched into his spiel: "I will be calling on each of you by name, so I want to spend a few minutes having each of you introduce yourselves. One thing you will discover about me is that I expect to pronounce each of your names correctly, just as I expect you to pronounce all words correctly." He pointed to me. "Apps," I said.

"You sure that's the correct pronunciation?"

"Yes," I said. No one had ever questioned how I pronounced my name before. After all, the name had been in the family for a long time, and I had never heard anyone pronounce it any other way.

He went around the room, hearing the students call out their names: Burmeister, Anderson, Caldwell, Williams, Miller..., checking them off in a little book he carried.

"This semester," he continued, pronouncing his words very clearly and distinctly, "we will be reading and analyzing *A Tale of Two Cities* by Charles Dickens." He was waving a copy of *A Tale of Two Cities* like a preacher waving a Bible. He was clearly into Dickens. I wanted to ask if we'd be doing any creative writing, but I thought better of it.

When English class met again, on Wednesday, the burly professor once again called off our names: "Adams, Anderson, Apps"—except he pronounced mine with a long *a*, "Apes." I corrected him. "Oh, yes, Apps," he blustered. So much for making sure all names and words were pronounced correctly. He never did get my name right, for the entire semester.

I don't know if it was true, but I later heard that this particular professor had no love or respect for agriculture students. Whenever we turned in an assignment, always something we'd written about *A Tale of Two Cities,* he would tear apart the writing. Not once did he offer a word of praise for anything I had written. I didn't know it at the time, but the best I could hope for in the course was a C. And that was what I got. I nearly gave up my love for writing because of this professor. Throughout the rest of my undergraduate years, my writing consisted only of required assignments—well researched, usually, but bland and, I must say, boring in style. Nothing creative or special.

But I can't deny that my first-semester English professor enhanced my vocabulary and improved my basic writing skills. I hadn't realized how limited my vocabulary was until I heard him speak. At times it seemed I couldn't understand a third of the words he used. I'd jot them down and after class look them up in the dictionary. I greatly improved my grammatical and analytical skills that semester too. In that introductory English course, we spent hours dissecting and analyzing *A Tale of Two Cities.* At the time I was more interested in improving my own writing skills than examining some-one else's, but the exercise forced me to learn how to take apart a piece of writing and look for its meaning at several levels. I learned one other important lesson that semester: just because you don't like a teacher doesn't mean you can't learn from him or her. In the end I learned much from this pompous character who insisted on calling me by a name that wasn't mine and caused a chuckle from my fellow classmates each time he called the class roll.

In contrast, I greatly enjoyed my agriculture courses and the professors, who were all former farm boys and understood country kids like me. The agriculture courses seemed more practical as well, including ideas that could be applied on the farm, such as what variety of alfalfa does best on which kinds of soil, how much lime to apply when your soil tests acidic, and how to adjust a tractor-pulled plow so it will turn a furrow just so. (I hadn't yet come to appreciate that courses that seemed impractical to me, such as chemistry and English, offered learning opportunities beyond immediate application, including critical thinking, problem solving, and an opportunity to view a broader, more expansive perspective on things.)

As the first weeks of the first semester flew by, I began to make some new friends, mostly fellow students in my agriculture classes. Courtney Swertz, Hubert Jorns, and Robert Kimball were farm boys too, and we had lots in common as we struggled with living in the city and adjusting to the University of Wisconsin. I also exchanged letters with a girlfriend back home, a high school sophomore whom I had taken to my senior prom, but since both my studies and a lack of extra money kept me from returning home on weekends, we slowly drifted apart.

By late September the nights had gotten cooler, and I began eating breakfast in my room because now I could keep a quart of milk on the windowsill and a package of sweet rolls in a dresser drawer. For lunch I purchased a summer sausage log, which I also kept on the windowsill, and a loaf of bread. I figured I could afford one meal a day at Rennebohm's or at the university cafeteria on Breese Terrace, as long I didn't pay more than seventy-five cents for it.

On a Friday afternoon a month after school began, I climbed on a Greyhound bus for my first visit home since going off to Madison. The bus dropped me off in Plainfield, about fifteen miles from our farm, where Pa picked me up. It sure was good to see him. Although he didn't say much, I guessed he was feeling good about seeing me too from the smile on his face. As we drove toward home, Pa asked me what I was learning at the university. I told him how among other things I had learned how to adjust a tractor-pulled plow and would be glad to help him adjust the plow at home. This proved to be a mistake.

Pa and I worked for more than an hour adjusting our David Bradley two-bottom plow so it would do a better job trailing behind the Farmall H tractor. As we drove the tractor and the newly adjusted plow to the already-harvested cornfield, I had high hopes for an improved performance. It didn't happen. The plow would scarcely turn a furrow without the soil falling back into place. Pa didn't say much of anything as we adjusted the plow back to where it had been. I learned a valuable lesson that day, one that farmers have said time and again: Book learning doesn't work all the time. I appreciated that Pa allowed me to try a new approach, even if it didn't work. It was another valuable lesson, one that had always been my pa's approach to things: Don't be afraid to try something new. If it doesn't work, at least you know one more thing not to try.

That first weekend home reminded me how much I missed the country. The trees in our woodlot were ablaze with fall colors: reds, yellows, several shades of brown. Pa had been cutting corn with the corn binder, and I spent a half day helping him stand the corn bundles into shocks that at day's end reminded me of a row of Indian tepees. The rich, musky smell of newly cut corn mixed with the subtle smells of newly turned soil where we had been plowing. The deep-blue sky contrasted with the goldenrods, the trees, and the green alfalfa pasture where our herd of black-and-white Holsteins grazed. What in the world was I doing cooped up in a little room on Orchard Street in Madison, with the noxious sounds and smells of the city all around me? I didn't share these doubts with my family, but I felt them as strongly that weekend as I ever would.

Back in Madison, the six-week examinations were drawing near. It was a dreaded weeding-out time in those days, for after the exams a good number of students would leave the university, never to return. I did well on the tests for my agriculture courses and earned a C in English, but I was close to flunking chemistry with a D. I had never gotten a D in twelve years of schooling. My other grades were good enough to keep me from being expelled or placed on academic probation. But how could I tell anyone that I had gotten a D in my first six weeks at the university, when I was supposedly the top student in my high school class? I felt like quitting and returning to the farm, but I knew I couldn't do that either. What an embarrassment that would be to my folks and to my high school teachers at Wild Rose.

That midway point of my first semester was probably my hardest time at the university. I was struggling with my bad leg, I was still spending three hours a week in the Red Gym pool, and what was I going to do about chemistry? I knew there would be more chemistry to come in my agriculture curriculum and more science courses that depended on a good foundation in chemistry. Still, I was grateful I hadn't been asked to leave the university because of low grades, which had happened to several students. I could just see the headline: Wild Rose High Valedictorian Flunks Out of University.

# 18   Paying My Way

On top of my other worries that fall, I quickly realized that the $150 in my checking account was not going to last for the school year. I asked Professor Bucholtz about any moneymaking opportunities he might know about. He introduced me to Professor D. C. Smith, chair of the Agronomy Department, who told me about an opening in the department's seeds laboratory. After a brief interview with Professor Smith, he told me I was hired. I would earn fifty cents an hour helping with research projects, and best of all, I could choose the times I would work. The following Monday afternoon after my classes I walked to the seeds lab, just beyond the old horse barn on the far west end of the campus.

My job turned out to be counting seeds for germination tests—one hundred seeds of one crop or another, mostly bromegrass seeds. The UW's agronomy professors and their graduate students were attempting to come up with more nutritious and higher-yielding bromegrass varieties and were testing several candidates. One characteristic they wanted information about was germination rates—what percentage of the bromegrass seeds planted would grow.

It was precise and painstaking work. I spread a bunch of threshed bromegrass material over a glass plate with a light beneath it. Then, peering at the grassy mixture, I looked for the little dark spot characteristic of bromegrass; the other stuff on the plate was chaff left over from the threshing process. With a pair of tweezers I carefully picked out the seeds from the chaff, counting out exactly 100 of them. Not 103, as I once did; not 98, which I did another time. An eagle-eyed graduate student was checking up on me.

After I counted the seeds I spread them in petri dishes and made sure they were properly labeled. Graduate students added water and a growing mixture and put the seeds in a warm place to germinate. After several days, I opened the petri dishes and counted the number of seeds that had sprouted. Eighty seeds sprouted meant 80 percent germination.

Besides earning fifty cents an hour, I learned two important lessons at that job. First, when doing research, attention to detail and accuracy are of vital importance. And second, it's best to learn to deal with mind-numbing boredom—life is full of it, as I would discover.

To add to my income, I picked up odd jobs on weekends. A bulletin board at the housing office listed local residents looking for students to help with odd jobs. One of the most interesting I found was helping a local doctor take in his dock on nearby Lake Mendota. He handed me a big wrench and asked me to loosen several bolts holding up the end of the dock. The bolts were rusty, and before you could say, "Make sure you've got a good hold of that wrench," I dropped the wrench in the lake and it sank out of sight in the mud. I was sure I'd be fired right there on the spot. But the doctor didn't fire me; he found another wrench, and after considerable effort I managed to loosen the bolts so we could pull the dock on shore for winter storage. It took most of the morning; I earned two dollars.

As I stuffed the dollar bills in my pocket, he asked me if I could return the following Saturday. His big home on the lake was a couple miles from Orchard Street, but I hoofed it over there the next Saturday and every Saturday morning the rest of that fall. He had all kinds of "make-work" jobs for me: I painted a big bird cage yellow with a tooth brush (this took me two hours). I polished all of his and his wife's shoes every Saturday morning, even though they hadn't worn them during the week. I was too dumb to realize it, but the doctor felt sorry for this skinny little farm boy with a limp and wanted me to have a little extra money. I surely needed every penny I could chuck in my pocket.

In addition to my Saturday morning jobs, one of the fellows in my rooming house had lined up some Saturday afternoon jobs and asked if I could help him. "Of course," I said. Together we put up I don't know how many storm windows that fall, many on three-story houses. One of the strangest jobs we did was painting the fire escape on one of the big office buildings on the Capitol Square for fifty cents an hour. We painted it using small paint brushes—my partner said using a small brush would make the job last longer. He was right; it took the two of us four hours to complete the job.

Too soon fall turned to winter, snow began to fall, and the outdoor jobs disappeared—except for snow shovel-ing, and I was not at all keen on doing that, especially with my bum leg. All the odd jobs I had done that fall had provided enough money so I could eat at least one meal a day away from my room. As for a social life, I essentially had none. In 1951 the lower limit for beer drinking in Wisconsin was eighteen, and on Saturday evenings the taverns around campus were filled with students. But I wasn't among them, for two reasons: I had no money, and I was only seventeen years old.

By the end of the fall semester, although I wasn't flunking out, I still wasn't doing nearly as well as I wanted. My grade point average for the first semester was 2.65, not even a B average. Of course, although nobody told me as much, I had spent most of the semester doing remedial work, particularly in chemistry. I had asked one of the chemistry graduate student teaching assistants for help, and he had walked me through the basics. I earned a C in my first course in chemistry and was happy with the grade, considering that I was doing both high school and college chemistry at the same time.

Before the beginning of the second semester, I changed advisors. I met with Walter Bjoraker, a professor in the Department of Agricultural Education, who agreed to work with me on my desired major, ag education. Walt, a Minnesota farm boy, smoked a pipe, was a little on the plump side, and was one of the most caring persons I ever met. He helped me map out the courses I would need to take to prepare me for teaching high school agriculture. He also boosted my rather low opinion of my first-semester grades when he said they were quite good considering that I had come from a small, rural high school. "The smaller schools often don't have strong college preparation courses," he said.

I didn't want to say anything negative about my high school, as I was quite proud of the place, and I knew I had gained skills there that would serve me well, such as writing and speaking skills and working with others to do quality work and meet deadlines, as we had on the school newspaper.

I was happy to return home during winter break. I discovered that my folks had purchased a TV set, and my brothers were staying up until ten each evening to watch programs. (I had gotten quite accustomed to indoor plumbing, but although our farm now had electricity, my parents hadn't yet installed indoor plumbing.) As we had done during Christmas breaks for as long as I could remember, my dad and brothers and I went ice fishing on Mt. Morris Lake nearly every day after the chores were done, sitting in a little fishing shanty heated with a woodstove and listening to uncles and neighbors spin stories. It was wonderful. Occasionally someone asked me about life at the university, and I told them it wasn't too bad. By the end of Christmas break I was actually looking forward to returning to Madison. Despite the difficulty of some of my courses (chemistry in particular), I had begun to enjoy the place.

The second semester went by quickly, with few problems. Chemistry 1b, while challenging, was much easier than the Chemistry 1a had been. My second-semester English course was more interesting too, although we spent more time reading and discussing books than writing, which is what I preferred to do. I had passed the swimming test in early December, so my regular dips in the chilly Red Gym pool were history. And I had gained a few more friends: Don Schwarz, John Cain, and several others. I got to know Jim Marcks, who I noticed walked with crutches with big braces on his legs. He told me that he had had polio when he was a kid. I had told no one about my polio experience, and I didn't tell Jim why I limped;

my problems seemed like nothing compared to what he was experiencing. About the only good thing about Jim's condition was that he was excused from both ROTC and physical education. He worked his way up and down the many steps and hills of the university's sprawling campus, never complaining, studying hard and setting the academic pace for his fellow students, me included.

By the middle of the second semester, I was no longer the lonely, limping freshman who was startled and confused by a big university and city life. And then, in the blink of an eye, the second semester was over and I was back home on the farm—out of money and already looking forward to the fall term.

It felt wonderful to be back on the farm again, helping with haying season, even hoeing cucumbers, potatoes, and green beans. I savored the sun on my back, the smell of freshly turned soil, a cloudless sky, bird song, and the quiet. Oh, how I enjoyed the quiet.

But now I had three whole months to earn money for the following school year. I heard that the California Packing Company in Markesan, about fifty miles south of Wild Rose, was hiring men for the pea harvest. By mid-June I was living in a dormitory fifty yards or so from the big canning factory, working mostly in the warehouse, where I stacked hundreds, maybe thousands, of cases of freshly canned peas. I was only seventeen, so it wasn't legal for me to work around machines. (Of course, as a farm kid I had been working around machines since I was little, but as the cannery manager said, "Rules are rules.") I was back to doing work that was mind-numbingly dull, requiring only a strong back and the ability to follow the foreman's instructions: "Pile these thirty cases over here, pile those fifty cases over there." Still, I was pleased to find that my gimpy leg handled the work quite well. The only good thing about the job was the pay: a dollar an hour, twice as much as I had made at any of my jobs in Madison.

In mid-July, as the pea-canning season was ending, George Luedtke stopped by the farm to talk with me. George, who had purchased my Grandfather Witt's farm after World War II, also worked as the manager of the H. J. Heinz pickle factory (more accurately called a cucumber salting station). At H. J. Heinz, workers received, sorted, and dumped cucumbers into huge silo-like tanks with salt and water added to cure them.

George had a little mustache that jiggled up and down when he talked. "Jerry," he said, "would you like to take over my summer job as manager of the Heinz pickle factory? I think you'd be good at it."

I was tempted to say that I was just a limping farm kid with no experience managing anything—I had difficulty managing myself. But I didn't. I asked what was involved. George explained how the factory worked. I knew some of what he was telling me, as we had hauled cucumbers to the Heinz factory as long as I could remember, and I had watched what happened to our cucumbers once they were dumped into the sorter. He told me the hours would be long, starting at eight in the morning and going on until the last cucumber was dumped into a vat. "In mid-season that usually means after midnight," George said. But then he added, "The pay is pretty fair; as manager you'd get $1.25 an hour. Oh, and Monica Etheridge is our bookkeeper. She keeps track of the payroll, keeps all the records, writes the checks for the cucumbers purchased, and figures the salt. She's worked several summers and knows the operation well."

"Figures the salt?" I asked.

"Heinz is fussy about how much salt and how much water go in every tank. Monica keeps all that straight so you don't have to worry about it."

George must have put in more than a good word for me, because without being interviewed or even filling out an application, I got the job. I was the new manager of the pickle factory. But I had one problem. The cucumber season began around the middle of July, and I couldn't go on the payroll until I turned eighteen, on July 25. So for the first week—which I mostly spent getting acquainted with everything and working alongside George—I received no pay. George hired the work crew that summer, which consisted of Monica Etheridge, Bernie Van Airsdale, Alson Attoe, Vernon Huber, and Junior Jones, who had recently been fired from his job at the local sawmill because of a drinking problem. Bernie and Alson were high-school-age tough guys who knew how to work but didn't get along well with each other. Vernon was probably in his fifties and a hard worker, and Junior, in his forties, worked hard when he was sober. Monica, who spent most of her time in the pickle factory's makeshift office—it did have a door that closed—was the only woman on the crew.

Day and night we sorted and salted cucumbers, hundreds of bushels of them. We sorted the cucumbers into five grades, from the smallest "number ones," called gherkins, to the jumbo "number fives." All went into the big wooden tanks with salt and water. We worked seven days a week, usually shutting down the sorter sometime after midnight and starting things up again shortly after eight in the morning when the first cukes began arriving. In those days nearly every farmer in this part of

Waushara County raised from a quarter acre to an acre of cucumbers as a cash crop.

One big commercial grower, Jim Burns of Almond, had more than a hundred acres of cucumbers. They were picked by migrant workers of Mexican heritage who came north from south Texas to work in the cucumber fields of central Wisconsin. Every day Burns's foreman and several of the workers delivered a couple of truck loads heaped high with burlap bags of cucumbers. We talked with them, joked with them, and even learned several cuss words in Spanish. It was my first contact with Spanish-speaking people.

Although I continued to limp and sometimes tripped over things, my bad leg mostly served me well at the pickle factory that summer. The hard work of lifting and moving thousands of pounds of cucumbers strengthened my arms and back, and it helped my legs as well. As long as I didn't have to run, I was in good shape.

By the end of August, thanks to my jobs at the pea cannery and the pickle factory I had saved enough money for tuition, clothes, rent, and food to take me to at least Christmastime. I spent a few days helping Pa fill our silo, and I was once more on my way to Madison. To save my money for the year ahead, I hitchhiked, something quite easily accomplished in those days. All of my possessions easily fit in one medium-size suitcase. Pa drove me to Highway 51, which ran through Plainfield, and I thumbed my way back to Madison and another school year.

# 19   Sophomore Year

I was happy to return to my little room on Orchard Street, which I had come to love. (In fact, I stayed in the same room all four of my years at the university.) To save money, I kept my routine of eating breakfast (usually a sweet roll or two and a glass of milk) and lunch (a couple of slabs of summer sausage on dark bread and another glass of milk) in my room. For supper I headed either to Rennebohm's or to the Breese Terrace Cafeteria, where I usually ate alone with my nose in a book or sometimes with one of the other students from my rooming house. There was nothing fancy about either eating place, and nothing fancy about the food either. I usually ordered some kind of casserole and always spent less than seventy-five cents. I was skinny as a rail but, as some of my farm friends would say, healthy as an ox. Indeed, I don't recall missing one day of school in four years because of illness.

My courses in my sophomore year were more interesting than the required freshman-year classes had been. During the first semester in 1952, I took sixteen credits: zoology (1), dairy husbandry (1), agriculture economics (4), agricultural engineering (9), and agricultural education (1). Of course, I also signed up for my

Receipts for my first-semester sophomore-year tuition and textbooks

required ROTC class, for which we earned no credits. I found the ROTC air science courses to be considerably boring because most of the instructors knew not a whit about how to teach.

We wore uniforms to ROTC classes—leftover army officer uniforms with air force patches on the sleeves. The United States Air Force had separated from the US Army in 1947, but we continued wearing the old army uniforms called pinks and greens—the pants were pale gray heavy wool (some said with a hint of pink) and the coats dark brown (not at all green). Under the coat we wore a tan shirt and brown tie. The uniforms were hot and uncomfortable, especially at the start of the school year before the weather turned cooler.

Our ROTC training included marching—learning how to stay in step and how to keep a cadence, which was called by an ROTC instructor: "Hup-2–3-4, hup-2–3-4." We learned how to do turns and turnarounds, in unison, without tripping and bumping into each other. We must have been quite a sight to see on those first days when we were learning the army way to move from one place to another.

During my free time I worked at the seed laboratory, but I was becoming more and more bored with counting bromegrass seed (and now Sudan grass seed) into one-hundred-unit lots. The friend I had worked with painting fire escapes and putting up storm windows said he'd heard of a job in the music school that might be more exciting than counting seeds for germination tests. The

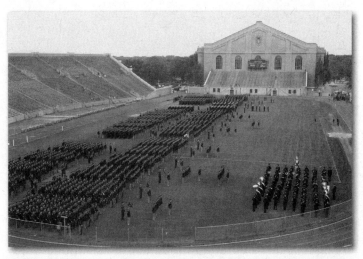

ROTC training included marching—lots of it. We marched in parades, including a Memorial Day parade down State Street in Madison. We also "passed in review" while marching in Camp Randall Stadium, as seen in this 1952 photo. We spent many hours in the classroom as well, learning how to be military officers. *WHi Image ID 75915*

pay was the same, fifty cents an hour, but it included evening and weekend shifts, so I could accumulate more hours. He suggested I make an appointment to see Professor S. T. Burns, the head of the music school.

I met with Professor Burns at his office in Music Hall on the east end of campus. After a half-hour discussion, it seemed that Professor Burns was going to trust me to be in charge of the music school's practice rooms, which were located in a three-story building across Park Street from Music Hall. My job would also include setting up the stage in Music Hall for the university orchestra's performances. I told Professor Burns that I didn't know how to set up for an orchestra (at the time I didn't know the

THE UNIVERSITY OF WISCONSIN
COLLEGE OF AGRICULTURE

Madison 6

DEPARTMENT OF AGRICULTURAL EDUCATION

February 6, 1953

To the Assignment Committee:

Jerald W. Apps, an advisee of mine, finds it necessary to carry a job while in school. He is currently employed by Professor Smith in Agronomy and it is quite necessary that he have Friday afternoons open. We would appreciate it if you could arrange his schedule to permit this and in addition, it would be highly desirable if Mondays and Wednesdays from 3:30 on could be left free.

Walter T. Bjoraker
Walter T. Bjoraker
Assistant Professor
Dept. of Agricultural Education

b/mf

In the second semester I requested a change in my academic schedule so I would have time to work at my new job in the music school—and be freed from counting seeds in the Agronomy Department.

difference between a bassoon and a French horn). He said that someone would teach me. He didn't even ask if I was a music student—I guess he'd figured that out from my comment about bassoons and French horns.

He did ask me where I was from.

"Wild Rose," I answered.

"I know where that is," he said. "Up there in the center part of the state."

I nodded.

"Can you start tomorrow?"

"I can," I said, smiling. "I'll be here around three, after classes."

"Good. Stop here, and my secretary will give you the rundown on what to do, along with the keys you'll need."

I had a new job, and it seemed I had one more person looking out for me, helping me stay in college. I hadn't mentioned polio, and Professor Burns hadn't asked about my gimpy right leg. When I thought about how easy it had been to get the job, it occurred to me that Professor Burns had a difficult task finding a student who was willing to work every evening and on weekends. Most students wanted time off for doing a little partying, for dating and having a social life. My social life at the time consisted of chatting with students between classes. No partying, no dating—I simply didn't have enough money to do anything beyond what was needed to stay in school.

Thanks to my lack of a social life, I was able to work thirty to forty hours each week at the music school, on top of going to school full-time. I earned twenty dollars a week. But the job was more than a good source of income. It was interesting—far more so than counting seeds. I had a tiny office tucked under the stairway of the practice hall, a three-story building with small practice rooms on each floor. My main tasks were to schedule the rooms for one-hour practice sessions for music students, to lock up at night, to open and close the place on weekends, and to generally keep order, as Professor Burns described it. About once a week I had to set up the stage in Music Hall for the orchestra.

Students signed up for hour-long practice sessions, usually a day or so in advance. Some students signed up for at least an hour every day, so I soon got to know them well. I had never known musicians before other than our guitar-strumming hired man back home. I discovered that the music students were a likeable bunch, friendly and easy to get along with—mostly. When they learned that I wasn't enrolled in the music school, they somehow

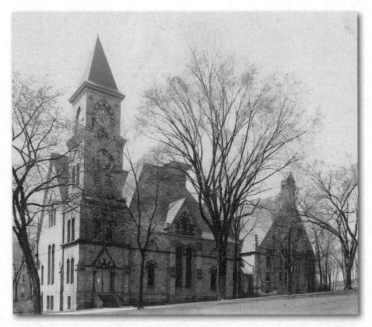

I spent many hours working in Music Hall for fifty cents an hour, the standard wage for student workers at the time. *WHi Image ID 58025*

decided I was a good person to listen to their problems and concerns. I heard about their boyfriend/girlfriend problems, their unhappiness with certain music school instructors, their worries about being drafted into the military, everything. They trusted me not to share any of what they told me, and I never did.

Imagine the sounds in that practice hall, which had no sound proofing: a piano in one room, a violin in another, a trumpet blaring in still another, a vocalist trying to hit a high note, a saxophone going to it—all at the same time. In between sign-up times, which happened once each hour, I could spend the time studying. Slowly I developed the ability to tune out all the noise (and noise it was, far from music). Soon I was doing all of my studying at my noisy little office.

I did have one other responsibility. The music school had a strict rule against smoking in the building, a rule I was supposed to enforce. And, as Professor Burns had pointed out to me, the practice rooms were for practicing music; no other kind of practice, such as getting better acquainted with a girl- or boyfriend, was appropriate. And so once an hour I patrolled the halls, stopping in front of every closed door, listening and smelling. If I smelled smoke, I knocked and reminded the culprit of the no-smoking rule; if I heard no sounds I gently knocked and then entered to see what was going on. Occasionally I discovered a pair of embarrassed music students making a different kind of music. I referred to this part of my responsibility as my "smoking and smooching" patrol, which most of the music students found quite hilarious. In my nearly three years working there, I busted no more than a dozen students for violating one or both of these rules. I never reported anyone—such a report would have banned them from the building. I simply reminded them of the rules. I was just eighteen years old the first year I worked there, and every music student was older than me, but nobody asked me my age. Nobody cared. We all got along fine.

In the second semester of my sophomore year, the war in Korea continued raging. The next summer, on July 27, 1953, the United States, North Korea, and Russia would sign an armistice to end the war. But of course in the spring of 1953, no one knew how long the war would go on. That spring I would finish my second year of required ROTC classes. Not enrolling in advanced ROTC would mean becoming eligible for the draft, so I signed up to take the advanced course for Air Force ROTC in the fall with high hopes of becoming a jet fighter pilot when I graduated. However, it was not to be.

The advanced military programs required a physical examination before acceptance. I was told to report for my physical to Madison's Truax Field, an active air force base at the time, where a team of air force doctors and technicians gave me the once over. No one asked me if I had had any diseases such as polio, and I didn't offer the information. The medical team seemed much more concerned about my eyes than my legs. This was the first time I had had an eye examination, and it was a doozy. It took most of the afternoon to complete. The results: an air force doctor said, rather bluntly, "In a couple years you'll be wearing glasses. Our pilots must have perfect vision." (He was right. Within five years I was wearing glasses.)

Now I was stuck. I needed to be in some kind of advanced ROTC program to keep my draft status so I could stay in college, so I immediately applied to Army ROTC.

They cared not a whit about my eyesight. Nor did they inquire about my having had polio, or much of anything else.

"What do you want: infantry, military police, signal corps, transportation corps?" a clerk at the Army ROTC office inquired. Transportation corps sounded interesting; I had no desire to be a frontline infantry officer, didn't care much about policing, and didn't know anything about the signal corps. So I enrolled in the Transportation Corps ROTC, with advanced courses beginning in the fall term of 1953, when I would be a junior.

As soon as school was out that spring, I spent a week at home, helping Pa and my brothers with haying. By the end of June I was back working at the pea cannery in Markesan, only now I was eighteen and could work around machinery, so I was promoted to viner boss. I would earn $1.25 an hour.

Each of the canning companies in those days owned several stationary pea viners, machines that separated the peas from the rest of the plant (today's pea viners are portable and work directly in the fields). The viners were scattered around the countryside, sometimes several miles from the cannery in Markesan. A stationary pea viner somewhat resembled a grain threshing machine, about ten feet tall and twenty feet long. A huge turning cylinder with holes in it did the work of separating the vines from the peas. A worker forked the heavy, often tangled vines onto an elevator that fed the material into the machine. The peas came out the bottom and were captured in wooden boxes; the empty pods and pea plants were elevated onto a stack where another worker forked them into a reasonable pile. The green pea vines fermented in the pile, making pea silage, which area farmers hauled back to their farms and fed to their cattle in winter. While the pea silage was fermenting, or "working," a foul-smelling, fly-drawing liquid trickled out of the bottom of the stack. It was something no one wanted to step in, yet we often did, because it was always there.

The work crew I supervised that summer included a high school teacher from Markesan, a sensible and good worker probably in his forties; a fellow from Jamaica who spoke with an interesting accent and worked hard with nary a complaint; a farm boy my age who said little but knew how to pitch tangled pea vines; and a man in his early fifties, rather frail, who was drunk by midafternoon almost every day. We rotated the work as the day wore on: two guys pitched peas into the viner from the pile the farmers dumped on a little platform every hour or so, one fellow worked on the stack, one fellow took the peas from the machine and put them on a scale, and I weighed each box of peas and recorded the information so the farmers could be paid the correct amount for their crop. I also was in charge of keeping the machine running. I gassed up its Farmall M tractor engine every morning, and the machine didn't shut down until all the pea vines the farmers had delivered had been processed, usually around midnight or one in the morning. We worked from 6:00 a.m. to the wee hours of the following morning, seven days a week. The only time we had to rest was when it rained, which it did only two or three times during the six weeks of pea harvest.

By the second week on the job, I decided I had to find the liquor bottle that I knew must be hidden somewhere near the pea viner. I couldn't have a drunk crew member working around the machine—he might fall into it and be maimed or even killed. So I kept the man working on the stack, away from the machine. But almost every day he fell off the stack and into the ooze of slimy, smelly, greenish liquid that trickled from the fermenting peas. He was a smelly mess—liquor mixed with pea vine ooze—and nobody wanted to be anywhere near him. Finally one day I shut down the machine and the rest of us searched for his bottle—and found it. As he watched with an astonished look on his face, I poured the booze on the ground. We all went back to work, and I had no problems with the fellow for the rest of the pea harvesting season.

With all the work experience I had accumulated, I was more relaxed and sure of myself that summer. As soon as the pea season was over, I was back in Wild Rose managing the H. J. Heinz Pickle Factory with the same crew I had the previous year. It was a good cucumber-growing year, and we were busy seven days a week, usually late into the night, receiving, grading, weighing, and dumping cucumbers into the big tanks with the appropriate amounts of salt and water.

Once again my summer passed in a haze of hard physical work. Working off the farm earned me many times more than I could have earned growing cucumbers and beans at home or doing farmwork as a hired hand. No one limited the number of hours we could work in a day in those days, and an average day of sorting pickles or pitching pea vines was often sixteen hours—at $1.25 an hour I was pulling in twenty dollars a day. I was pleased that as a manager I earned more than the workers.

Being manager had another benefit—one I never mentioned to anyone. It allowed me to avoid some of the most difficult and physically challenging jobs that I knew would tax my bad leg beyond its limits. Unloading a railroad boxcar of bulk salt with a long-handled shovel was about the most miserable, backbreaking job in the pickle factory. I didn't have to do it. By this time I had learned the physical limits of my polio leg, and other than becoming tired, it served me well, to the point that nobody seemed to care that I limped a little. I suspect everyone was so tired by late in the evening that they simply didn't notice.

As I look back on my summer jobs, I realize I learned much more than I understood at the time. Those summer jobs taught me about diversity, human relations, and how to get along with a bunch of guys who sometimes had trouble getting along with each other, especially when they were tired. Fights were not uncommon, sometimes turning into wrestling, hitting matches. Somehow I learned how to stop guys from killing each other. I did not have much of a physical presence—I was only five foot nine inches tall and weighed no more than 165 pounds. So I had only words to use in breaking up several heated confrontations over the course of the summer. Maybe I was just lucky, but no one at either the pea viner or the pickle factory started a fight with me. I guess they knew I would fire them on the spot if they did.

Summer work kept me too busy to do any writing beyond the reports I had to submit to the pea cannery in Markesan and to H. J. Heinz in Portage. But I was gaining an understanding of character, how working-class people interacted, the words they used and how they used them, their actions and reactions to situations. Without my realizing it, all of those firsthand experiences found a resting place in my memory and would be invaluable to me later as I developed as a writer.

# 20    Final University Years

I had been looking forward to my junior year, as it meant I was more than halfway to completing my degree. My dad always said that the second half of a trip seems shorter than the first half. He was right.

When I returned to Madison that fall, I was as comfortable as I'd ever been as a college student. I knew the ways of the university, knew how to work my way through registration, and for once wasn't worried about running out of money. I returned to my job in the music school and to my single room on Orchard Street (still five dollars a week). Now that I was enrolled in advanced Transportation Corps ROTC I even received a small government stipend, around twenty-five dollars a month. I continued doing most of my studying while at my music school job. I was paid fifty cents an hour to study—how blessed I was.

My course work now related to my major, agricultural education. One class required that I practice-teach vocational agriculture at an area high school. (I would have to successfully complete five weeks of practice-teaching at five different high schools during my junior and senior years.) In midsemester, a friend dropped me off on a Sunday night at a rooming house in Mount Horeb, about twenty miles southwest of Madison. The rooming house was within easy walking distance of the high school where I was to practice-teach for the coming week. I was more than a little scared; I had just turned nineteen in July, so I knew that some of the high school students would be almost as old as I was. Would they listen to me? I'd heard horror stories about what students did to practice-teachers. I slept little that Sunday night, thinking I'd rather face a half dozen coarse-talking, hardworking pickle factory workers than a classroom of high school students.

The next morning I met Mr. Johnson, the vocational agriculture teacher at Mount Horeb High School, who said I should observe him teach the first day. On Tuesday, I could take over the freshman class, and by Friday, if everything went well, I could teach all four classes. I discovered a great group of farm kids, and in the end my age worked to my advantage—I could see myself sitting in their seats just a few brief years earlier. They listened, they smiled at my lame jokes, and most importantly, they behaved. I wore a necktie every day, which seemed to give me a little authority—at least it seemed so to me.

My grades had improved considerably from that miserable first semester of my freshman year when I didn't know if I would make it or not. In fact, by spring semester of my junior year I was invited to join Alpha Zeta, a national honorary agricultural fraternity, which required a 3.25 overall grade point average.

That spring I also joined Delta Theta Sigma, a social fraternity for agriculture majors. I participated in the foolishness of the initiation process, which was supposedly top secret and not to be shared with anyone, and became an active member. I knew most of the members from classes we attended together. I was invited to live at the Delta Theta Sigma house, but I declined; I'd found I could do my best writing and thinking in my room on Orchard Street, with no one else around. Because I worked every night and every weekend, I never attended the fraternity's Monday night meetings, never ate at the frat house, and attended none of the social events. Why the fraternity put up with me, I will never know.

Advanced ROTC required all cadets to attend six weeks of summer camp between the junior and senior years of college. "Summer camp" was a euphemism for army basic training, six of the most grueling, difficult weeks I have ever spent. I arrived at nine-thousand-acre Fort Eustis a week after school was out. Nearly nine hundred ROTC officer cadets from across the country converged at this army post on the James River in Tidewater, Virginia, not far from Williamsburg. I was assigned to the first platoon of Company C—about forty of us from around the country, including several from Wisconsin.

Army basic training would be one of the most severe tests of my bad leg yet. Because I had been doing lots of walking all year and was otherwise in relatively good shape, I found I could compete with my fellow cadets reasonably well, except when running was involved. I was able to keep up when we jogged—called double time in the military—and thankfully we weren't asked to do any running beyond that. We started every day with physical training (PT), which involved push-ups, sit-ups, jogging in place, squat jumps—the kind of activity

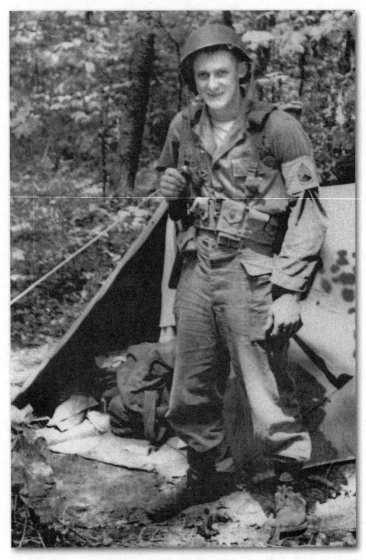

During the summer of 1954 I completed my basic military training at Fort Eustis, Virginia. Here I am as an acting sergeant, on bivouac at Camp A. P. Hill in the "wilds" of northern Virginia.

that benefited my bad leg while strengthening my good leg and my arms and shoulders so I could "cover" for my bad leg when necessary.

The six-week routine included too many hours of mind-numbing classes covering everything from the trajectory of bullets to how to read a map, from military history (not much) to what to do during a gas attack. We also learned how to make a "military bed," meaning we used hospital corners to keep blankets and sheets in place, and stretched the top blanket so tight that a quarter would bounce when tossed on it. The outdoors training was more interesting, and sometimes more challenging, for my gimpy leg. We spent several days on the firing range. Unlike my fellow cadets from cities like New York and Philadelphia who had never touched a gun, I had fired a rifle since I was eight or nine years old. As potential army officers, we were trained to use .30 caliber carbines and .45 caliber pistols, plus introductory training with .50 caliber machine guns, bazookas (anti-tank weapons), hand grenades, and mines (we laid out a mock mine field).

With my carbine, I shot at targets on the firing range, sitting, standing, and prone. I found it to be a fun couple of days away from a stuffy classroom and doing something I already knew a good deal about. The .45 caliber pistol was a different matter. When a rifle fires, it kicks back against your shoulder. A large-caliber pistol, such as a Colt .45, jumps in your hand every time you fire it, making aiming a considerable challenge.

I didn't realize it at the time, but ROTC summer camp had an important function besides training us to become soldiers and officers. It was designed to weed out those who could not physically or mentally adjust to army life. By the end of the second week, two or three cots were empty in our barracks as cadets had washed out—we never found out the reasons, except for one chap in our platoon who had a nervous breakdown. He simply couldn't adjust to a schedule where everyone did everything at the same time, every day except Sunday.

During the sixth week of basic training, we faced the biggest challenge of all, both physically and mentally. It took place in a huge field of bare ground—red clay that created a fine red dust when dry and when wet became the most challenging mud I had ever known. Tangles of barbed wire attached to wooden frames were spread randomly around the field. Every twenty yards or so, also randomly placed, were craters filled with water. And the most frightening of all: .50 caliber machine guns stood at one end of the field, designed to fire about thirty inches above the ground with live ammunition. The drill instructors warned us that the bullets were real and if anyone stood up the machine-gun fire would cut him in two. We had already learned from other cadets that the situation was as close to real combat conditions as possible.

To add to the stress and difficulty of the course, the exercise was conducted at night—a very dark night, as it turned out. A half dozen or so of us maneuvered through the course at one time, crawling while carrying our carbines in front of us. Sometimes we moved on our backs to work our way through the barbwire, but we usually were on our bellies, using our elbows to propel us along. The machine guns pounded away, sending tracer bullets over our heads. Tracer bullets look like menacing fireflies, and you can see the bullets as well as hear them whizzing overhead. Having spent more than five weeks being challenged in every possible way, I wasn't about to let this exercise unnerve me—but it almost did. I made the mistake of crawling too close to one of the water-filled craters. Those craters had explosives buried in them—explosives that the drill master occasionally set off as cadets neared them. When I was within a few yards of it, I heard an enormous explosion, and red mud nearly buried me. I couldn't see and my ears were ringing from the concussion of the explosion. I rubbed the mud out of my eyes, made sure I had my carbine securely in hand, and continued crawling toward the end of the course, which had to be no more than one hundred yards of misery ahead. I looked back to see a cadet who had apparently given up. He was lying still. I hoped that he hadn't lost it and decided to stand up. Not long after, I wiggled through the last barbwire entanglement—I was blessed to have had lots of experience with barbwire on the home farm—and met the drill instructor, who told me I had passed the course. In fact, I was one of the first to complete the course. Obviously my arms and shoulders, which had done most of the work, had served me well.

I had successfully done what some polio-free cadets were not able to do: I had made it through the rigorous and mentally challenging training and had excelled at times. The longstanding feelings of worthlessness that had plagued me since I had had polio were at their lowest ebb in years.

With six weeks of army basic training behind me, I returned to Wild Rose and managed the Heinz pickle factory for rest of the summer. I was in great physical condition for the pickle factory's long and often arduous work. My leg felt the best it had in years, I suspect because all the muscles around those that had been affected by the disease had been working overtime.

Then it was back to college for one more year of courses and practice-teaching (three weeks in three different schools). I continued working at the music school, often forty hours a week, and with the money from my summer work, the ROTC stipend, and a hundred-dollar scholarship from the College of Agriculture, I was able to save enough money to buy a car, a 1949 V8 Ford coupe I purchased from my cousin, Barbara Jean Witt, for three hundred dollars. To keep my expenses low so I could afford gas, I continued living in my little room on Orchard Street, where the rent was still five dollars a week, and I still ate breakfast and lunch in my room. I did occasionally break my rule of not spending more than seventy-five cents for an evening meal, although I didn't have much time to eat anyway, as I could not be away from my little desk alongside the stairway in the practice hall for any length of time.

Now that I had my Ford, I did manage a few dates. For a time I dated a girl from Lake Geneva who lived in a privately run all-girls home on Langdon Street. The woman who owned the place ran it like an overprotective mother—all the girls had to be in by ten on weeknights and midnight on Fridays and Saturdays. She stood at the door when the girls returned, checking them in and giving dirty looks to their dates, me included.

The early 1950s was mostly a quiet and serious time on campus. Many older and married veterans were still attending classes, and they wanted nothing to do with the foolishness that some younger students organized. The goofiest episodes were panty raids, when male students tried to steal coed's undergarments by invading the girls' dormitories. Of course the coeds cooperated, often opening windows to allow male students to enter or even saving them the effort by tossing unmentionables out the windows. It was a prank that spread across college campuses at the time, perhaps in the same category as swallowing goldfish or trying to fit as many students as possible into a phone booth. My work schedule precluded such activity—and besides, I had worked too hard to earn my college degree to chance being arrested by a campus cop for stealing girls' underwear.

I studied hard, worked hard, marched a lot (ROTC cadets did a lot of marching), and soon it was graduation weekend. I had learned that I would be graduating with honors and was invited to the Honors Convocation held in the Memorial Union the day before graduation. I was one of eighteen College of Agriculture students graduating with honors. I so wished that my mother and dad and brothers could have attended, but chores on the farm took precedence. I think my folks would have been proud, because the entire family had worked hard to make sure that I could graduate from college—I was the first one even in the extended family to earn a college degree.

The convocation was the first time I had heard President Fred speak since he welcomed us to campus four years earlier. His comments were brief:

*Congratulations, Distinguished Scholars of the Class of 1955.*

*We honor you today for your splendid scholarship. We are grateful for what you have given the University and your classmates while you have been making the most of the academic opportunities at the University of Wisconsin.*

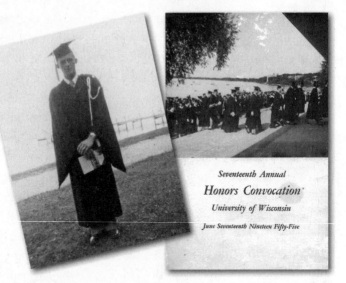

Seventeenth Annual
*Honors Convocation*
University of Wisconsin
June Seventeenth Nineteen Fifty-Five

*(top left)* I was the first in my family to attend college, and my graduation from the University of Wisconsin was a proud day for all of us. *(top right)* I attended the Honors Convocation as part of my graduation ceremonies. I wished my folks could have been there, but doing the farm chores took precedence.

> *It is our confident belief that you who have led your classes will continue to be leaders in the building of a useful life. Informed citizens, who will contribute generously in time and energy, are our nation's best hope for building a better world.*
>
> *Our best wishes are extended to each of you for a life filled with success and happiness.*

Mother and dad and my brothers did make it to the commissioning ceremony on Saturday morning, when all the ROTC seniors received their commissions as second lieutenants in the US Army Reserve. We all wore our uniforms, of course, and we nearly filled the football stadium when we marched in, presented the colors, and stood at attention during the entire ceremony.

That afternoon, now wearing my cap and gown, I marched across the stage and received my diploma from President Fred. For once I was not at all ashamed that I limped a little on my way to shake President Fred's hand and receive my diploma with the other members of the class of 1955.

I had two letters to answer, one from the North Carolina State College of Agriculture and Engineering in Raleigh and another from the New York State College of Agriculture at Cornell University. North Carolina State had invited me to enroll in their graduate program in agricultural economics, with an assistantship that paid $1,800 a year. Cornell University suggested I enroll in their graduate program in rural sociology with an assistantship of $1,600 per year plus full tuition. Both were wonderful opportunities, but I had to turn them down. The US Army had dibs on me for the next six years.

# 21    Waiting to Serve

After graduation I worked on the home farm until the
pickle factory opened in late July. I learned I would be
the factory's last manager. At the end of the summer H. J.
Heinz closed the place, and after the cured cucumbers
were moved to Pittsburg the following spring, the company sold the building and the tanks.

With the pickle factory closed, I returned to farmwork, helping with the fall harvest, filling silo, and cutting the last crop of hay. When hunting season opened
I hunted squirrels and rabbits, pheasants and ducks.
My twin brothers had graduated from high school that
spring, and Donald was home as well. He was on a waiting list to enter barber school in Eau Claire, and that fall
we worked and hunted together. Darrel was a freshman
at the University of Wisconsin in Madison. In October
Don and I, and the neighbor boys, Jim and Dave Kolka,
took a job raking cranberries in a cranberry marsh near
Wisconsin Rapids. We worked in rows of several men
strung across the width of the marsh, raking cranberries
by hand for eight or nine hours a day, wading in frigid
water, always trying to keep up with the man working to
our right. It was hard, backbreaking work. At the pickle

factory, I had been the manager and could decide what I did and how I did it. In the cranberry marsh, somebody else made all the decisions, and I was a common laborer, earning about a dollar an hour.

It was a strange time for me. I had a degree from the university, I was certified to teach high school vocational agriculture and biology, I had two offers to do graduate work in study areas I enjoyed, I was a commissioned officer in the US Army—and I was doing common labor. Nothing wrong with common labor, of course, but I had expected something different. I was sure that no high school would hire me as a teacher when they learned that in a few months I would be on active duty in the military, so I didn't even bother to apply.

As I labored in the cranberry marsh that fall, I was still waiting for my orders from the army. I expected two years of active duty somewhere in the world. The Korean War had ended in 1953, but I assumed I would be sent to Korea to be a part of the peacekeeping action following the war. Of course, I would go wherever my orders instructed me.

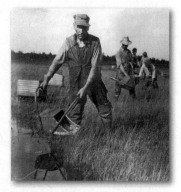

Finally in late October my orders arrived. After three months of advanced training at Fort Eustis, I would serve two years in

Like the men in this photo, I raked cranberries by hand from early morning to near dark.
*WHi Image ID 1874*

Germany. I was elated. My grandmother Apps was from Germany, and both my great-grandparents on my mother's side had come from that country. In a strange kind of way I felt I was going home. But most importantly, now I could make plans for the future. I sold my 1949 Ford to my brother Donald, along with some of my clothes.

With the cranberry work completed, Don and I hunted, ice fished, and generally had a good time that fall and early winter as I waited to leave for Germany and he waited to enter barber college. The day after Christmas I got a phone call from George Collum, the depot agent in Wild Rose.

"I've got a telegram for you from the army. Just came in, but it's got lots of letters and numbers that I don't understand. Suppose you could come down and help me figure out what it says?"

I drove down to the depot, and together George and I deciphered the telegram. It was a change in orders. I was not going to Germany. I was still supposed to report to Fort Eustis, on January 16, 1956, but I was to enroll in the Transportation Officers Basic Course (TOBC) for three months, serve an additional three months with a training unit at Fort Eustis, and then come home. Then I was to serve five and a half years in the active reserve, attend weekend meetings, plus participate in two weeks of summer camp each year. The telegram didn't say this, but newly minted second lieutenants were in oversupply at the time, and with the Korean War over, the army was cutting back its active-duty force.

I was both disappointed and happy. I had been looking forward to spending some time in Germany at the government's expense. But now I could find a teaching job as early as the fall of 1956. On January 13, along with four other second lieutenants, I was on my way to Virginia—a long drive, as there were no interstate highways then other than the Pennsylvania Turnpike.

The morning after we arrived at Fort Eustis I met the formidable First Lieutenant Half. He was but one rank above me and my fellow second lieutenants, but you'd think he was a general the way he lorded over us and ordered us around. I suspect some of us were a bit cocky, being junior officers and all, and needed to be brought down a peg or two. Lieutenant Half was just the one to do it, and he began on that first day.

As transportation officers, we learned how to load cargo ships, working as stevedores for a week. We loaded railroad cars, we loaded cargo airplanes, we learned the capacities of various motor vehicles and helicopters, we learned how to drive diesel locomotives, we drove semitractors with loaded trailers (I discovered that the shifting gear on the semi-tractor was the same configuration as the shifting gear on our Farmall H tractor, so I had no problem), and we learned how many combat soldiers could be packed into a landing craft (the only combat unit in the transportation corps consisted of those who drove landing crafts). And we did physical training every morning, without fail. We marched in parades every Saturday, rain or shine. Compared to Wisconsin, the weather in Tidewater was unbelievable. The morning temperatures that January seldom reached as low as 32 degrees; in the afternoon it sometimes got into the low 70s. The hard work I had done in the cranberry marshes the previous fall, and all the hiking my brother and I did while we hunted, had served my gimpy leg well. It was as strong then as it would ever be, although my limp was still noticeable, especially after a long day of training.

When the three-month training program ended, my fellow officers and I were assigned to various units at Fort Eustis. I was assigned to the 507th Transportation

Battalion (Movement Control). Our job was to figure out how to move people and equipment from here to there. One of our tasks that summer was to assist in the loading of cargo ships headed for Hudson Bay for the DEW (Distance Early Warning) Line radar sites that were being constructed across Canada. Construction had started in December 1954 and would continue until the sites were operational on July 31, 1957. The transportation corps's sizeable fleet of small cargo ships could quite easily navigate in relatively small places, such as into Hudson Bay from Hudson Strait.

During active duty my battalion had more officers than work to do. I often completed my work by early afternoon and would head to the PX to have coffee and shoot the breeze with my fellow underemployed officers. But more often I would just drink coffee by myself and think about my future. I decided that spending day after day, year after year, in the same high school classroom was not something I wanted to do. I liked being outside. I liked doing a variety of things. But I also liked teaching. I mulled this over, wondering how I could teach, particularly ag topics, but not do it in a high school classroom.

As the days slowly passed, I also thought about the decision I had made when I started college to keep my humble beginnings under wraps. I had begun to understand that I should be proud of my upbringing rather than ashamed of it, that my experiences growing up provided me with a personal history that I could use in whatever career path I decided to follow. Growing up on a farm had surely helped me during my time in the army: I'd been shooting a rifle since I was ten years old; I had no fear of the outdoors—indeed, I preferred being outside to inside; I adjusted easily to the primitive condi-

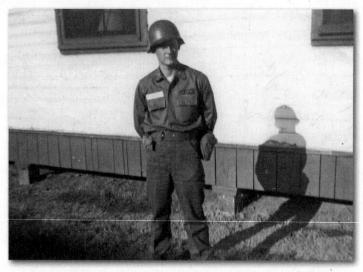

As a second lieutenant on active duty, I was stationed at Fort Eustis, Virginia, where I was placed in the transportation corps, the army unit responsible for hauling everything from soldiers to ammunition.

tions we faced on army training missions, having grown up with few conveniences. My early experiences on the farm clearly compensated for my gimpy leg caused by polio. I began to envision a career working with farm families, helping them improve their lot, accept their background, and understand that who they are and what they do as farmers was as important as any other profession—perhaps even more important.

When I completed my active duty in mid-July, I was finally free to find work, to return to graduate school, or to do whatever I wanted as long as I attended regular reserve meetings and two-week summer camps for the remaining five and a half years of my six-year commitment. I also learned that it was possible to complete correspondence study in lieu of attending reserve meetings. I returned home and spent the rest of the summer working for my cousin, Vernon Apps, who managed a cucumber receiving station in Wild Rose for the Chicago Pickle Company.

After my time in the army, I knew what I wanted to do with my life. Working in agriculture was on the top of the list. In fall I enrolled in the graduate school at the University of Wisconsin–Madison, with a research assistantship in the Department of Agricultural and Extension Education. The assistantship paid me for working half-time on a research project that would result in a Master of Science thesis. Dr. George Sledge, a recent graduate of Michigan State University, was my advisor.

In my four years in the undergraduate program, my writing had suffered terribly. I had completed the necessary term papers for my college courses and had done well on essay examinations, but because of the bad experience I had in college English courses, I wasn't at all sure of my writing abilities. I had done almost no creative writing since leaving high school. Now, for the first time in nearly five years, I was writing again, and feeling good about it. But I definitely felt rusty. Five years is a long time to be away from something.

I discovered that I enjoyed graduate school a great deal. Even though I was working half-time on a department research project, I still had time to think, to write, and to meet many interesting people. I made many new friends, including Helgi Austman, an agricultural extension worker from Winnipeg, Canada, and Arthur Brehm, an extension agent from Dodge County. During our noon lunch breaks we played poker using paper clips as chips (the department had an unwritten rule against playing cards for money). About once a week we settled up, turning paper clips into pennies. Art Brehm still owes me $1.49 cents in poker winnings.

About a dozen of us grad students, men and women, had desks in a huge, windowless, fourth-floor room in Agriculture Hall, a place that had once housed white rats and guinea pigs used by the Bacteriology Department. One of the grad students was a square-dance caller, and about two nights a week, after we had studied for an hour or so, we square-danced. What fun we had. I had never square-danced before, but even with my gimpy leg I discovered that I could do it. Even better, I learned how to call square dances, a skill that I enjoyed tremendously and that I would later put to good use as a county extension agent.

Nearly all of my new friends were extension employees from someplace in the world. When I had decided I didn't want to teach high school agriculture but still wanted to work with rural people, I hadn't been sure what career to pursue. Now I was introduced to the idea of becoming an extension agent. My graduate courses in animal science, agricultural journalism, and particularly a course titled Introduction to Extension (taught by Professor James Duncan, a former extension agent himself), were of great interest to me. For these courses I could include a bit of creativity in my writing assignments, which helped remove some of the rust from my long-ignored creative writing skills.

I completed my master's degree in record time—two semesters—and was quickly on the job market. In April 1957 I interviewed in Green Lake County and received an offer to become the county's 4-H agent, part of the field staff of the UW College of Agriculture's Cooperative Extension Service. My annual salary was $4,600—an enormous amount of money, I thought, compared to my income from various part-time jobs and my salary as an army officer. Nevertheless, when the agricultural and extension committee of the Green Lake County Board interviewed me, one of its members let me know in no uncertain terms that just because I had a master's degree, I shouldn't expect any more money in my pay envelope. He wanted the job done; he cared not at all about advanced training or degrees. (Green Lake County contributed one hundred dollars a month toward my salary; the remainder came from state and federal sources.)

My office was in the basement of the courthouse in downtown Green Lake, where I worked with G. Willys Gjermundson, county agricultural agent, and LaVerne Priebe, county home agent, to provide out-of-school educational opportunities for the rural families in Green Lake County—farmers, homemakers, and children.

When I arrived at the Green Lake County Extension Office at 7:30 on Monday morning, June 17, Willie Gjermundson was already behind his desk. "Welcome to Green Lake County," he said. "We're all going to the 4-H camp at Patrick's Lake in Adams County for the annual spring cleanup day." By "all" he meant himself, LaVerne, and me, plus several Green Lake County 4-H leaders. In July Green Lake County 4-H members would be spending a week at Patrick's Lake. 4-H groups from several other counties in the region also camped at Patrick's Lake, and they all shared the task of keeping the place in tip-top shape.

The camp was about an hour's drive west of Green Lake, on a little hill above Patrick's Lake, a small, shallow body of water that was spring fed, with no inlet or outlet. I later learned that the Patrick's Lake 4-H camp had been a Civilian Conservation Corps camp that operated during the Depression. It had closed down during World War II and then reopened as a 4-H camp. It was quite primitive, at least by today's standards, comprising two bunk houses (one for boys and one for girls), a dining room–kitchen building, two outhouses (girls' and boys'), and a hand pump that stood between the bunkhouses and the dining room. The place had electricity but no indoor plumbing, and the camp cook prepared meals on a wood- and coal-burning cookstove.

My fellow Green Lake County Extension staff members and I traveled west through Princeton, Harrisville, and Westfield and then into Adams County to reach Patrick's Lake. Ten volunteer 4-H leaders were already there to help us with the cleanup. When we arrived, Willie told us the jobs to be done: sweeping out the bunkhouses, washing the windows, cleaning the kitchen, dusting and cleaning everything in the dining hall, and digging new pits for the outdoor privies. I volunteered to dig the privy pits. Later I thought about the irony of that: less than a year earlier I had finished a tour of duty as a second lieutenant in the army; a few days ago I had completed a master's degree at the University of Wisconsin; and here I was shoveling out a toilet pit, a job I had done several times at the home farm when I was a kid. Though I didn't know it at the time, because I was content to dig a toilet pit on my first day as an extension agent, the volunteer 4-H leaders saw me as an ordinary guy who wasn't afraid to get his hands dirty. That would serve me well in my job, as I would work with many of them during my years as a 4-H agent. There was (and still is) a feeling on the part of some people that those of us with college degrees lack practical skills and ideas. The old saw "Too much book learnin' can spoil a person" hasn't completely faded.

Years later, when I think about my writing, I often think of my first day on the job as a "professional educator," digging privy pits in Adams County. A writer knows that for one's ideas to be accepted, the listener or reader has to first accept the person. From the time I completed active duty in the army, my goal was to work with rural people—to write material that they could read and enjoy and, I hoped, learn from—and give talks that they would find both entertaining and informative. I learned to avoid writing (or talking) down to people and trying to impress them with high-flown words, long complicated sentences, and meandering paragraphs that sounded good—writing that might impress another educator but that would leave an audience saying, "Huh? What's this guy trying to say?"

A particular skill is required in using a shovel to dig a hole. Likewise, a particular skill is needed to write something that an audience of country people will appreciate and learn from. I have worked at improving these writing skills for more than fifty years, and I have a long way to go. Someone asked me once how I learned to write. I responded, "I haven't learned how to do it yet. I'm still working on it—and I suspect if I ever get it figured out, that's when I'll quit." I'm a firm believer that all of us, no matter how skilled or accomplished we may think we are, still have much to learn.

After my first day at work at my new job, I returned to my rooming house in Green Lake more tired than I'd been since my days working at the pickle factory and the pea cannery. But it was a good tired, and my bad leg had come through with flying colors.

While I was in Green Lake County, I began writing a weekly column for the Berlin and Green Lake newspapers titled "Four-H News." The column was part of my professional responsibilities, but I had creative leeway to tell stories about what I had observed the previous week, introducing an interesting person, sharing a historical fact I had uncovered, and of course promoting Green Lake County's 4-H program. It seemed the more creative I was in my writing, the more favorable the comments I received from my readers.

Before long I was doing a weekly live radio show for WCWC, a radio station in Ripon that covered our area. The station had come on the air just a few weeks before I started my new job, and a station representative visited our Green Lake Extension Office to inquire if Willy, LaVerne, or I would be interested in having a regular radio program. I volunteered, and soon I was on the air sharing stories about Green Lake farmers, tidbits of history, even some practical information for 4-H members ("Here are some tips for preparing your calf for the fair"). The feedback from listeners was most encouraging (although some of the comments had nothing to do with what I was talking about, such as "Gee, you have a good radio voice"). Some folks thanked me for taking time to "talk with them on the radio."

In lieu of attending regular army weekend drill sessions, I enrolled in the Army Transportation School's Extension Program and was completing weekly lessons by mail on such topics as "Leadership," "The Transportation Corps in Army Aviation," "Military Passenger Movements," "Beach and Inland Waterway Operations," and more. I had to attend a two-week summer camp each year as part of my military obligation, and that first summer I traveled to Camp McCoy, near Sparta, Wisconsin, where I was attached to a transportation unit. They didn't know what to do with me. Along with a captain from Minnesota, I was told to spend the two weeks traveling around the camp and evaluating the activities. We both knew our assignment was "make-work," but we took it seriously. On some days, we would park our jeep on top of a hill and watch the troops march or work on the firing range. We also drank a lot of coffee those two weeks. At the end of our stint I wrote a "comprehensive report," using as much creativity as I thought I could get away with. When the captain and I filed our report, the officer in charge of the unit was most impressed with what we had to say about his unit and thanked us for making him and his troops look good.

In October 1959, my second year working in Green Lake County, I attended a district extension meeting in

Portage. There I met Ruth Olson, who was working then as a temporary home economics agent in Sauk County. I thought she was the most attractive woman in the room, and I knew I had to get to know her better. But district meetings in those days were all business, and about the only conversation I could manage was a hello and a mention that I worked as a 4-H agent in Green Lake County. Ruth said she had just been hired as a permanent home economics agent in Waushara County, where she would start on November 15.

I got to know Ruth better during the extension's annual conference in Madison later that month. County extension workers from all over the state gathered in Madison for a week of updates from extension specialists, inspirational talks from Cooperative Extension Director Henry Ahlgren, and socializing in the evening. The single agents gathered each evening at the Idle-Hour Bar on the east side of Madison, as far from campus as we could get. There Ruth and I had a chance to chat, enjoy a beer or two (Ruth came from a teetotaling family, so beer drinking was a new experience for her), and get better acquainted.

We both were busy with our jobs, but we managed to see each other from time to time. After she moved to Wautoma in November it was easier, since Green Lake and Waushara Counties are adjacent. One of our favorite outings were the dances at Lakeside Lodge, a popular polka dance hall on Fish Lake near Hancock. We must have been a sight to see: the limping German polka dancer and the good-looking blond Norwegian woman who was just learning the ways of the central Wisconsin polka dancers.

In January 1960 I started a new job as 4-H and livestock agent for Brown County, and I moved to Green Bay.

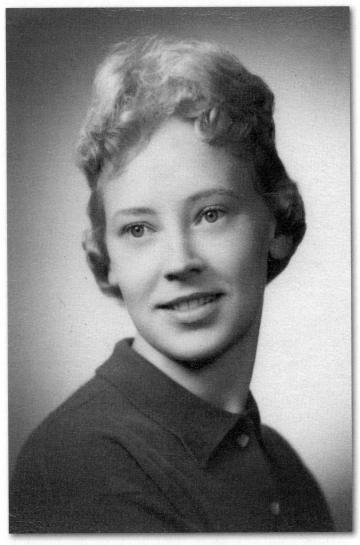

I met the lovely Ruth Olson when I was working as an extension agent in Green Lake County. She was about to start a job as a home economics agent in my home county of Waushara.

In 1960 Green Bay boasted three TV stations (WLUK, WBAY, and WFRV), plus several radio stations. In addition to the daily *Green Bay Press Gazette*, several Brown County communities had weekly newspapers. Soon I was writing two weekly columns, one for the *Press Gazette* and one for the weeklies. I also wrote a monthly newsletter that went out to several hundred farm families. I did one, sometimes two radio programs a week and one or two live TV shows a month. Ray Pagel, farm editor for the *Press Gazette*, was one of those crusty old newspaper editors I've come to appreciate and enjoy. By that time I thought I knew something about writing—apparently just enough for Ray to take me under his wing and give me weekly lessons on how to improve my columns. Orion Samuelson (now with WGN in Chicago) was farm director at WBAY-TV; from him I learned much about how to do live TV without making a fool of myself.

That same year I met Robert Gard. A Kansas farm boy with interests in writing, folklore, and drama, Bob did outreach work for the University of Wisconsin–Madison, helping local groups organize writing clubs, produce plays, and in general become more involved in the arts. I invited Bob to help with a drama workshop I had organized for the 4-H clubs in Brown County. It was a delightful day watching Bob teach the kids and their volunteer leaders the basics of drama. Bob's style was always encouraging, with little criticism, yet he was able to draw the best out of the youthful actors and actresses he worked with that day.

I managed to find time to travel to Wautoma every week or so to see Ruth, who was as busy as I was, helping homemaker groups and other rural women improve their lives. We were engaged on November 11 (Armistice Day,

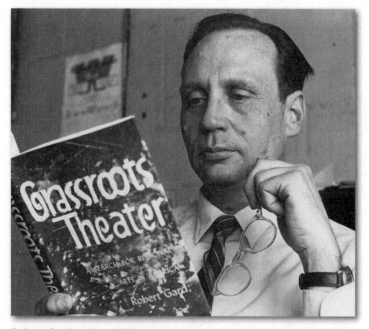

Robert Gard, author, folklorist, teacher—and my writing mentor for many years. *WHi Image ID 91338*

so we both had the day off), 1960. We set our wedding date for May 20, 1961—and then we barely saw each other before the wedding, as spring is a busy time for extension workers. The week before the wedding I was in prison— our extension office had an arrangement with the Green Bay Reformatory, which kept an outstanding dairy herd at the time. I conducted a dairy judging workshop for Brown County 4-H members at the prison on May 13.

Before we married I sold the little eight-by-twenty-four-foot trailer where I had been living since my days in Green Lake, and Ruth and I rented a bungalow at 1242 Cass Street in Green Bay. The proceeds from the sale of the trailer were enough for us to buy furniture for our new home.

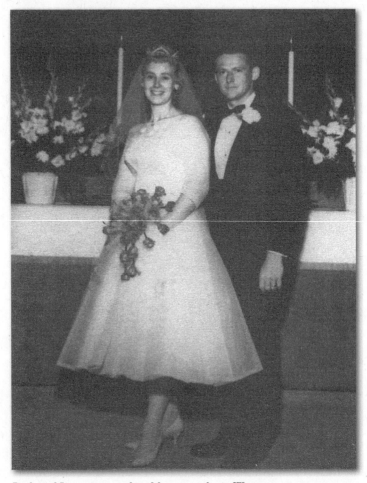

Ruth and I were married on May 20, 1961, in Wautoma.

In spring 1962 Frank Campbell, state 4-H leader, asked if I'd like to work as a publications editor for the state 4-H office in Madison. I would edit and write bulletins for 4-H members on topics ranging from forestry to dairy, from canning to clothing construction. I would also be responsible for organizing radio and TV programs for the state 4-H office and would meet with

4-H volunteer leader groups, giving talks at their annual recognition banquets held throughout the state. I was excited about the opportunity to do more writing and the challenge of becoming an editor, and after a lot of discussion, Ruth and I agreed I would take the job. Our daughter Susan was born in June 1962, and we moved to Madison in August so I could start my new position.

As extension agents we all held faculty positions in the College of Agriculture, and my new job included a promotion to assistant professor. Now I was writing and editing nearly full-time. My office staff consisted of a copyeditor, a designer, and a secretary. We were usually overwhelmed trying to keep up with the demands of the thousands of 4-H members around the state who depended on us to produce their educational materials. We did everything except the printing, which was done by the Agricultural Journalism Department staff on offset presses located in Hiram Smith Hall.

I did manage to find time to continue my own education, enrolling in an agricultural journalism course on editing taught by Lloyd Bostian. Hardly a day went by that I didn't apply in my professional work something I learned in the course. I had discovered that the previous two persons who held my position had been journalism majors. Since I had neither a journalism degree nor an English degree, this information did not help my inferiority complex, but it surely spurred me to learn as much as I could about nonfiction writing and editing.

By now I had worked six years for Cooperative Extension, the time when decisions are made about tenure. Soon I would be informed whether I could continue in my position with some job security or would have to find other work. Dr. Mitch Mackey, personnel director for Cooperative Extension, stopped by my office one day. "Jerry," he said, "it's time to gather your materials so we can put your case forward for tenure."

I was so busy writing and editing that I hadn't given any thought to tenure. "Do I have to?" I asked.

"You do if you want to keep working for us," he answered. He wasn't smiling when he said it. I quickly pulled together some of my writing—articles I had contributed to a national 4-H publication, newspaper columns and stories, plus a fistful of bulletins I had written or edited. I gave all of this to Dr. Mackey and forgot about it. A month or so later he stopped by my office. "You now have tenure, Jerry," he said. This time he was smiling. At the time I had no idea how important having tenure was.

In 1963 Professor Jim Duncan, who had been one of my instructors for my master's degree, received an invitation to teach at a newly formed agricultural university in Brazil. Walt Bjoraker, who now chaired the Department of Agricultural and Extension Education, asked if I would be interested in teaching Jim's course, Introduction to Extension, part-time.

I agreed, and I discovered that I enjoyed classroom teaching after all. I had taught a few workshops for Extension before, but in a semester-long course I could develop ideas in depth and get to know the students better. In 1964 I moved full-time into the Department of Agricultural and Extension Education, with a split appointment between campus teaching and Cooperative Extension. For Extension I would now focus on staff development, helping to improve and support the teaching activities of Cooperative Extension field staff. One of my assignments was to help develop "how-to-teach" materials for field staff. I also soon found myself writing budget narrative for the annual budget request materials that all university units had to submit each year.

I now had two bosses: Dr. Bjoraker in the ag department, and Dr. Patrick Boyle, head of the extension and staff development. I also had a mandate from Glen Pound, dean of the College of Agriculture—I must earn a PhD degree before I could be promoted to associate professor, and I would receive no salary increases until I did. By this time Ruth and I had two sons, Steve and Jeff, along with Susan—a fairly strong incentive to get that PhD.

I enrolled in the School of Education with a major in adult education and minor in rural sociology and immediately began taking one course a semester toward my degree, besides working full-time teaching and doing staff development work for the extension. In those days a reading knowledge of two foreign languages was required for a PhD, so I was soon studying French and then Spanish. Advanced courses in statistics were also required, along with several courses in research methods. It was a tough time for my family, as I had little time to be with the kids, who were four, three, and two at the time. "Where's Daddy?" was a question too often asked; I was locked in the bedroom with my head in an advanced statistics book or studying French or Spanish verb conjugation. I had to relearn (or learn for the first time) the nuances of English verb conjugation so I could make accurate translations to English, enlisting the help of my niece Janet Olson, a high school senior at the time. All of this has proved extremely helpful later when I began doing part-time and then full-time freelance writing.

By 1965 I had served the army in the reserves and on active duty for a total of ten years, and I received an honorary discharge. The army would have been happy to keep me, but with three young children, a full-time job, and my course work, it was time to leave something behind. Besides, the Vietnam War was now raging, and there was a good chance I would be called up for active duty.

In 1966 I went on leave from the university to complete the research for my PhD degree and write my dissertation on rural community leadership. It was the first time since 1957 that I could arrange my own schedule and work at my own pace, and the family appreciated that I had more time for them. The downside was that we had little money—my fellowship didn't come close to covering the expenses of a family of five, which included a monthly mortgage payment for a small home we had purchased on the west side of Madison a couple of years earlier. I did some freelance teaching for Volunteers in

## Honorable Discharge

from the Armed Forces of the United States of America

This is to certify that

JEROLD W APPS  04 057 323  Captain  Transportation Corps

was Honorably Discharged from the

## Army of the United States

on the 25th day of October 1966  This certificate is awarded as a testimonial of Honest and Faithful Service

RUSSELL S HESSE
CAPT  AGC

DD FORM 256A, 1 MAY 50

I received an honorary discharge from the US Army Reserve in 1965. I had reached the rank of captain.

Service to America (VISTA), a program created by the Lyndon Johnson War on Poverty legislation. But I spent most of my time working on my dissertation. In those days, PhD dissertations, especially in the UW–Madison School of Education, all fit within a rather cut-and-dried format—an approach that offered little leeway for someone who wanted to be a bit creative with his writing.

From Bob Gard, then a member of the Department of Agricultural and Extension Education, I learned about Al Nelson, a full-time Milwaukee-area writer and part-time writing instructor. I enrolled in one of Al's evening classes and learned how to find markets for freelance writing, how to write query letters to publishers, and how to submit articles for publication. I began mailing articles to publishers and collecting rejection letters. I've said I've been turned down by some of the finest publications in the United States, and it's true. *Reader's Digest*, the *New Yorker, Atlantic Monthly* all turned me down with nicely printed rejection forms: "Sorry, your submission does not meet our needs at this time. The Editors." Of all the articles I submitted, not one was accepted. Meanwhile, after attending one of Al Nelson's workshops with me, Ruth wrote an article about how to prepare venison and included several recipes. She didn't write a query letter. She didn't research possible publications. She sent her article to *Outdoor Life,* which I subscribed to at the time, and a few weeks later received a typed letter with an editor's signature and a check for seventy-five dollars.

"What's so difficult about getting published?" she asked. Meanwhile, my stack of rejection letters grew taller each week as I continued writing and submitting articles, nonfiction and fiction alike. I got into the routine of spending mornings working on my dissertation and afternoons writing articles and short stories. My afternoons made my mornings bearable.

In 1966 my brothers and I bought a small farm from my father for one dollar. It is just two miles away from the home farm, where my parents still lived at the time. Ruth and the kids and I camped at the farm that first summer in an old leaky tent while I began taking down the old barn, which was about to topple onto the granary. By late summer I was back in Madison, putting the finishing touches on my dissertation and continuing to freelance write. Now two of my interests, writing and the outdoors, came together again, just as they had when I competed in forensics in high school. I came up with the idea of writing a weekly newspaper column on happenings at our farm: my observations of the pond as the seasons changed, the wildflowers we were finding, the wild animals living on our property, songbirds we'd seen, and more. I called my column Outdoor Notebook. In early November 1966, I sent a few sample columns to the *Waushara Argus,* the weekly newspaper published in Wautoma that I had grown up with. A couple weeks later I met with Howard Sanstadt, editor of the *Argus,* who told me he would run the column for a few weeks and see what reaction it received. The first column ran later that month; the *Argus* paid me five dollars for it.

I was encouraged by the letters and comments my column evoked, and I was happy to no longer receive rejection letters. The column appeared every week; some were good, some not so good. Every Monday morning I had to have 500 to 750 words in the mail to the *Argus* (and by 1970 three other newspapers, all owned by the *Argus,* were running the column). Eventually I began including photos with the columns, taking and developing my own pictures. (The payment, however, remained at five dollars, even after the column appeared in four newspapers and included both written material and photos.)

In January 1967 I walked across the stage in the UW–Madison Fieldhouse and received my PhD degree. It was a proud moment for my entire family, who had sacrificed so much during the years that I had my nose in a book and had little time to be with them. My brother Darrel and his wife, Marilyn, held a reception for my family at their apartment near the Fieldhouse. They invited my major professor, Burton Kreitlow, to attend. My dad and mother were there, somewhat overwhelmed by all the pomp and circumstance of the PhD graduation ceremony, and I'm sure feeling a bit out of place. When Professor Kreitlow commented to my mother about how proud she must be that I had received a doctor's degree, her response was, "He's not really a doctor. He can't even cure a chicken." For my mother, who hadn't graduated from eighth grade, there were three kinds of doctors: veterinarians, medical doctors, and dentists. A PhD-type doctor didn't make the cut in her book.

True to his word, Dean Pound immediately increased my salary, and in the spring I was promoted to associate professor (two years later I would be promoted to full professor). Starting in the spring semester of 1967, I was back in the classroom and on the payroll again. I continued writing weekly columns, and that spring I shared some of them with Bob Gard, who graciously read them, offered a few comments, and encouraged me to keep going. That summer Bob, who was also the director of the School of the Arts in Rhinelander, a two-week workshop featuring all forms of writing as well as other arts such

Waushara Argus, Wautoma, Wis., Sept. 24, 1970 SECTION THREE

# The Country Is Its Own Teacher

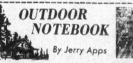

**OUTDOOR NOTEBOOK**

By Jerry Apps

Kids and the country go together well. That really isn't news to anybody. Except it really impressed me the days we were vacationing at Roshara. Our kids are city kids. They know about blocks, and sidewalks, and traffic. These they take for granted and have made a part of their lives.

So the country is new to them, a whole new set of experiences. There are no sidewalks at Roshara. A block is four miles around, and traffic--well every time a car goes by the farm we stretch our necks to see if we know who it is.

But there are much greater differences than the obvious. Take the day we were walking in the far corner of Roshara where there's a little woodlot--maybe a couple acres of black oak trees and some gray dogwood and hazel brush. Of course there's much more if you stop and look. That day we were doing lots of stopping and looking.

Susie saw it first. "What is it?" she asked as she pointed to the mound of dirt, punched full of holes on top and crawling with ants.

"It's an ant hill, Sue. Let's watch it for awhile,' I suggested. Sue and Jeff wanted to get as close as they could and before they were aware, ants were crawling over their shoes and then on their bare .legs.

"Dad, dad, there're on me!" Sue screamed. Jeff didn't say anything, he just jumped up and down and shook all over. I helped brush off the ants and then we sat down and talked about the ant hill, the society ants have, how they store food, and so on.

I'm sure both Sue and Jeff had read about ant hills in their school books, but until now an ant hill was some kind of abstract thing existing only on the dead pages of a book. Now they were learning about ant hills, by watching, by listening, and by feeling. The experience was real, alive to them. It just happened, it wasn't planned yet the children learned.

That same afternoon the kids were walking to the neighbors for some drinking water -- our well water is still questionable for drinking. On the driveway they found a small turtle -- and we nearly didn't get the water. The three of them spent most of the afternoon playing with the turtle. (They did stop long enough -- with some encouragement -- to bring back the jugs.)

What's so fascinating about a turtle? One lived in their aquarium at school. But this turtle was different. Here was a turtle all by itself, on the way to the pond I suppose, and the kids could pick it up and look at it. They could feel the turtle's leathery shell and watch its head slip in and out.

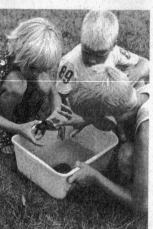

EXCITING DISCOVERY–It was only a little turtle, yet the kids were fascinated and played most of an afternoon with it.

They put the turtle in a pan with a stone and some water and watched it. They saw how it breathed, saw what it would do when turned on its back -- in a split second it was uprighted.

And then they had to make some decisions. What to do with the turtle? Keep it as a pet? They liked that idea. But I suggested we had no suitable place. Let it go? "But it's so much fun to play with," they cried.

The decision was finally made, they carried the turtle to the pond.

"He was goin' that way anyway," Jeff said. "This way he got there quicker."

You can't really teach kids about the country, you can only bring kids and the country together. The teaching will take care of itself.

## Mt. Morris

Mr. and Mrs. Ronald Leutner of Sleepy-eye, Minn. and Mr. and Mrs. Richard Busick and children Brenda, Kevin and Lori of Coon Rapids, Minn. were recent visitors at the Hiltman cottage on Porter's Lake.

I wrote my weekly column, Outdoor Notebook, from 1966 to 1976. I consider those years my writing apprenticeship.

as painting and dance, suggested I attend. The writing instructors that summer included Al Nelson, Kentucky writer Jesse Stuart, the poet Edna Meudt, outdoors writer Mel Ellis, August Derleth, and Bob Gard.

Derleth, a Wisconsin native, poet, nonfiction writer, and novelist, had written well over one hundred books by this time. He was crotchety, opinionated, pompous, and overbearing, and I learned a lot from him. I still have the notes from his workshop. Here's what he said about good fiction writing:

Involve the reader quickly

The story is the core of good fiction

Well-developed characters are important

Every detail should further the story

Simplicity in writing is important

Pay attention to the exact meaning of words

Don't worry about overuse of "said" when writing dialogue

Single most important rule for writers: Write!

Derleth discussed many other things during his session, including some of the realities of writing novels. He told us that his book *Wind Over Wisconsin* had sold thirteen thousand copies in twenty-eight years and had earned about $3,500. I appreciated knowing this, because so far my main writing income had come from my columns, a tidy total of $260 a year. No question about it: I would keep my day job.

Next I sat in Bob Gard's workshop on regional writing. There I learned that a regional writer is one with a strong sense of place, a writer who is influenced by where he lives and the connections he has with that place. I was writing about my farm in my weekly columns—I was doing exactly what Bob was talking about.

In early 1968, I gave twenty-five of my best columns to Bob and asked him, if I gathered a hundred or so of my columns, were they good enough to be published as a book? "Some good material here," he said, in his slow, Kansan way of speaking. "But a good book is usually more than a collection of columns. Use some of these ideas, but then write the book as a story—it's the story that makes a book work." Bob was harking back to what Derleth had said, that storytelling is at the heart of good writing, whether fiction or nonfiction.

"You also need a theme—something that ties the book together, something that makes the story work," Bob advised me.

In my spare time I began writing a book about our family's many adventures on our farm. I described our efforts to restore an old weather-worn granary into a livable cabin and our project planting several thousand red pines, our first efforts at forestry. I read my published columns over and over again, searching for ways of organizing the ideas into chapters for a book. I expanded on ideas that appeared in the columns and restructured them into a story format. I wrote stories about Ole Knutson, the retired Norwegian carpenter who helped us turn our old granary into a cabin; stories about camping under the shade of the willow trees that grew just to the west of the old farm buildings; stories of sleeping in our leaky old tent while thunderstorms threatened to blow it down, but never did; stories about tree planting and pond life and our country neighbors, especially Floyd Jeffers, a bachelor farmer who lived across the road from our farm.

By the end of 1968 I had completed a draft of the book—quite a good one, I believed. I asked Bob to read it, and a few weeks later I sat in his office, expecting a glowing report on the excellence of my work.

"Good start, Jerry," Bob began. "You need to do a little more work before it's ready for publication."

I had already revised the manuscript three or four times. What else could I do to it?

"That old black willow tree, Jerry—the one that you've made a character in your book."

"Yes," I said. I was very proud of my choice of a tree as a character.

"You really don't seem to know that old tree very well. I want to know how it looks in winter when the branches are bare. I want to know about the sounds in summer when you sit under it and the wind caresses the leaves. I want to know the smell of the bark and how it feels when you run your fingers over it."

I was crestfallen. I had thought my book was ready for publication. I had also thought it was the best I could possibly do. I was wrong, of course. I learned two lessons from Bob Gard that day. Along with the importance of using all your senses when writing, I learned that when you believe you have done your best work—writing, teaching, painting, carpentry work, whatever you do—you can always do better. I was reminded of what my dad had said many years earlier, about how I should always do the best I possibly could, no matter what the task. Most of us stop too soon, believing that we've done our best work. But if we are fortunate enough to have someone challenge us, we can almost always do better. We can go from good to great.

I continued to rework the manuscript according to Bob Gard's suggestions. I knew that Bob had started a small publishing house based in Madison, but I hadn't even hinted that I hoped Wisconsin House might publish my manuscript. When I showed the book to him again, he asked if he could publish it. I immediately said yes. And in the summer of 1970 my first book, *The Land Still Lives*, was published in hardcover and appeared in bookstores.

I was on my way to becoming a writer, with the humble realization that I must keep studying how to do it, keep pushing myself to do better, and continue listening to editors who have pushed me beyond being merely good. I have been writing books ever since.

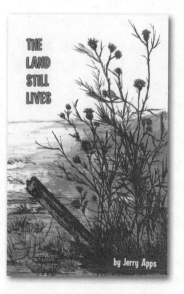

# Afterword

It was more than forty years ago that Wisconsin House published my first book. Whether he was aware of it or not, Bob Gard was my writing mentor on many book projects that followed.

In 1971 Bob asked me if I would be interested in teaching a class on article writing at the School of the Arts in Rhinelander. "Of course," I answered quickly. I went on to teach a variety of writing and book marketing classes at the School of the Arts for more than thirty years.

I continued writing my weekly column, Outdoor Notebook, until 1977. I produced 520 columns, never missing a deadline. I never earned more than five dollars for a column, so my total income for ten years of writing Outdoor Notebook was $2,600—not an earth-shaking sum. In 1973 I published my second book, *Cabin in the Country*, a collection of one hundred of what I considered my best columns. The book was published by the Argus Company, which also published the *Waushara Argus*, where my columns first appeared.

Ten years of weekly column writing served as my apprenticeship—my writing trial-and-error period. After the first year or so my editors gave me full rein to write whatever I wanted, following whatever style I wanted. When I messed up, they let me know. But they published my columns, the good, the bad, and the ugly. I made errors, lots of them. But I learned how to string together 750 words in such a way that usually made sense and evoked a response from readers.

During those years I also wrote articles, dozens of them; slowly editors began accepting and publishing them. I wrote on such things as how to make a bird feeder, round barns of Wisconsin, ice fishing, rabbit hunting, riding a bike to work, and more. My articles appeared in *Wisconsin Trails,* the *Milwaukee Journal,* the *Milwaukee Sentinel,* the *Capital Times,* the *Wisconsin Agriculturist,* and several other publications, earning me twenty-five dollars here, fifty dollars there, enough to keep me in paper and typewriter ribbon but not much more. I continued learning—and continued collecting rejection notices by the basketful. I tell my writing students that until they've collected enough rejection letters to cover the walls of their bedrooms, they've not completed their writing apprenticeship.

In 1977 I began working part-time as an acquisitions editor in the college division of the McGraw-Hill publishing company in New York. As an acquisitions editor, it was my job to locate authors and manuscripts related to college and university topics. I earned a yearly stipend plus a commission for each author and book I found, developed, and had accepted by the company for publication. About once a month I met with my boss in Manhattan at the McGraw-Hill building in Rockefeller Center. A highlight of those trips was lunch in the executive dining room on the fifty-first floor, with a panoramic view of the city.

In 1977, still teaching full-time at the University of Wisconsin–Madison, I began concentrating on book writing, now penning only the occasional article. I planned to write about one book every year or so. From 1977 to 1994 I wrote several books related to higher education, and I also wrote some about my first love, rural history and the environment. One of the most popular early books was *Barns of Wisconsin,* first published in 1977 and now in its third revised edition, published by the Wisconsin Historical Society Press.

I wrote my first novel in the late 1970s and had it accepted for publication by a regional publisher, along with a nonfiction book, *Breweries of Wisconsin.* The publisher ran into financial problems and published neither. *Breweries of Wisconsin* was finally published in 1992 by the University of Wisconsin Press. That early novel

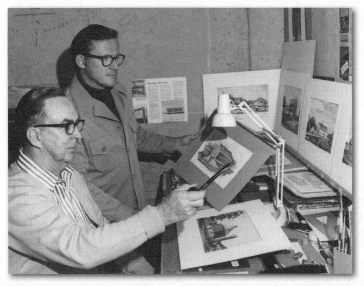

Illustrator Alan Strang and I reviewed artwork for *Barns of Wisconsin,* originally published in 1977.

rests quietly in a file in my office, never published. From the late 1970s until the mid-1990s, I had a series of literary agents. One gave up on me, I gave up on one, and a third—quite a good one—died. Since the mid-1990s I've marketed my own material to publishers.

By the late 1980s I had hoped to be writing full-time. Along with offering quiet words of support, Bob Gard made no bones about telling me to keep my day job. It was too risky to launch a full-time writing career and earn enough money to support a family, he said. I followed his advice for several more years. Bob died in 1997. I miss him.

I took early retirement from the University of Wisconsin in 1994, at age fifty-nine, finally ready to commit to writing full-time. By then our three children had graduated from college and were well established in their careers, and our family expenses were considerably less than when they were all in school. I enjoyed teaching, especially working with my graduate students. Less so did I enjoy administrative work; I had served seven years as chair of my university department, a challenging but often thankless job mired in reports, committee meetings, and personnel problems.

My love for nature is still at the heart of much of what I write. My feelings about the natural world run much deeper than merely appreciating its beauty. When I was recovering from polio and learning how to walk again, I often escaped to the woodlot behind our house. There, among the trees and emerging wildflowers, I felt accepted. It no longer mattered if I could walk or not. Nature offered comfort and acceptance, a place to think or not think, a place to recuperate and become restored.

When I was grieving the death of my mother and then my father, both in 1993, I found solace at my farm, sitting under a big oak tree overlooking my prairie, away from the clutter and bustle of the city, away from other people. For me nature is not only a place to enjoy but a place where I can quietly face challenges and problems. It also offers me an escape from my busy speaking and book-signing schedule. I enjoy being with people, interacting and sharing stories with them. But I also like being alone, finding a quiet spot where the phone doesn't ring constantly, where the only sounds are those of the wind and the wild creatures.

Since I began writing full-time in 1994, I have indeed published about one book a year, mostly nonfiction books for adults, but also four children's books and five novels. My speaking schedule is rigorous. With each new book, Ruth and I go on the road and I speak and sign books at libraries, historical societies, and bookstores in Wisconsin, Minnesota, Iowa, and occasionally Illinois and Michigan. I continue finding ways to combine

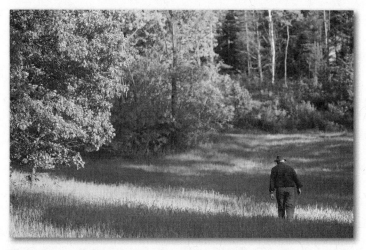

My farm provides me an escape, a place where I can be close to nature and where I can reconnect with who I am. *Photo by Steve Apps*

my three loves—writing, nature study, and public speaking—just as I did back in high school when I couldn't participate in baseball and basketball.

I continue to teach as well. I taught memoir writing for six years at the University of Wisconsin–Madison's weeklong Write by the Lake program, at the Green Lake Writers' Institute, and at Loras College in Dubuque, Iowa. In addition to my years teaching at the School of the Arts in Rhinelander, for more than twenty years I have taught at The Clearing in Door County, where I encourage students to write memoirs, reminiscences, children's books, novels, or whatever interests them in a workshop called Writing from Your Life.

When I reached the age of sixty, I began noticing that my limp was becoming more pronounced. Others noticed too. My polio leg that had served me well for so many years was rebelling. As each year passes, the limp becomes more noticeable, and walking has become difficult for me once more. It's called post-polio syndrome, when many of the symptoms that a polio victim first experienced return once more. Studies suggest that 25 to 40 percent of polio survivors experience post-polio syndrome, and the severity of the symptoms varies. There is little that can be done to treat it. But so far I'm able to write, speak, work on my forestry and prairie restoration projects, and garden. As long as my fingers work, my head is reasonably clear, and my voice remains strong, I will continue writing and speaking.

Polio is a dreadful disease. It maims and kills. Beyond its physical destruction, it has longtime psychological effects. I was fortunate; I survived the disease with only a gimpy right leg. The doctor who treated me said I was lucky to be alive. I suspect that was true, but being alive and not being able to do what other kids were doing at your age can be devastating. It can change how you see the world and how you react to it. I have never gotten over believing that I must constantly prove myself so I won't be seen as worthless. For indeed, worthless was how I felt for many years—and I suspect I still do to some extent today. As a result I have always worked hard, worked long hours, and, according to those around me, spent far too little time relaxing and enjoying myself.

Still, if I hadn't been stricken with polio as a child, I doubt I would have grown into the writer I am now. While my fellow high school students played basketball and baseball, I read books, studied, and wrote. Other than the writing dry spell of my college and early army years, I have been writing ever since. Writing is one of the most pleasurable, challenging, exciting, exasperating things I have ever done. Polio was no fun; post-polio syndrome is no fun either. Yet this awful disease is the reason I am writing today.

# Acknowledgment

Kate Thompson, senior editor at the Wisconsin Historical Society Press, encouraged me to do this project, as I had previously written little about my polio experience. Not only did she push me to do the book, she helped shape the project every step of the way. Thank you, Kate.

# About the Author

Jerry Apps has been a rural historian and environmental writer for more than forty years. He has published books on many rural topics, including *Every Farm Tells a Story, Living a Country Year, Rural Wisdom, When Chores Were Done, The Travels of Increase Joseph, In a Pickle, Cranberry Red, Tamarack River Ghost, Horse-Drawn Days,*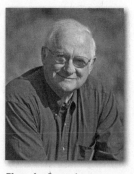

Photo by Steve Apps

*Garden Wisdom,* and *Old Farm.* He is a former county extension agent and professor at the University of Wisconsin College of Agricultural and Life Sciences. Jerry and his wife, Ruth, divide their time between their home in Madison and their farm, Roshara, west of Wild Rose—when they are not on the road.

*d*